BEYOND THE TURNOUTS

A COMPREHENSIVE GUIDE TO
FIREFIGHTER HEALTH & WELLNESS

JOHN HOFMAN JR.

CONTENTS

Preface v

1. Introduction 1

2. Overview of the Fire Service 5
   a. Cardiovascular: 6
   b. Strains and Sprains: 7
   c. Sleep: 9

3. Overview of Major Fire Services Wellness Initiatives 11
   a. NFPA Standards 12
   b. IAFF/IAFC Fire Service Joint Labor
      Wellness Fitness Initiatives (WFI): 12

4. Importance of Health and Wellness in the Fire Service 13
   a. Health Risks 15
   b. Cardiovascular Disease 15
   c. Hypertension 19
   d. Obesity 20
   e. Pulmonary Disease 21
   f. Cancer 22
   g. Joint and Back Problems 23

5. What Is Physical Fitness? 31
   a. Cardiovascular—Aerobic 34
   b. Cardiovascular—Anaerobic 35
   c. Muscular Strength 35
   d. Muscular Endurance 35
   e. Flexibility 35

6.   **How to Develop and Maintain Physical Fitness**...........................**39**

7.   **Nutrition**..**43**
    a. Fruits and Vegetables 43
    b. Carbohydrates 44
    c. Dietary Fats.. 44
    d. Proteins 45
    e. Vitamins and Minerals... 45
    f.   Water and Hydration 46
    g. Food Labels.. 50

Appendix A: Common Aerobic Exercise Equipment..........................**51**

Appendix B: Physical Assessments...**53**

Appendix C: Types of Aerobic Training **63**

Appendix D: IAFF / IAFC Candidate Physical Agility Test Preparation Guide..**65**

Appendix E: Training with a 48 / 96 shift schedule **69**

Appendix F: Example of a Dynamic Warm up..................................**73**

Appendix G: Determine your Target Heart Rate (THR).....................**75**

Appendix H: SMART Goal Setting: A Surefire Way
                     To Achieve Your Goals...**77**

References **99**

PREFACE

Fire suppression places a high amount of mental and physical stress on firefighters. Because these demands are so high, many fire recruits entering an academy are selected for their above-average physical fitness. Studies have shown that high levels of cardiovascular training, resistance training, and flexibility will reduce these risks and allow the firefighter to perform their skills more safely and effectively.

This manual focuses on current health and wellness risks in the fire service, corrective action measures to help overcome these issues, and education on improving one's overall lifestyle. In addition to, there are sample workout routines to improve cardiovascular training, resistance training, flexibility, and nutrition. By using this book, firefighters will be able to effectively:

- Evaluate their current level of physical fitness in order to monitor future progress

- Select exercise options that best meet their preferences, needs, and objectives

- Develop strategies and personal action plans that promote and improve total health and wellness

- Improve recovery time during post-fire ground operations

- Adopt a long-term commitment to a healthier physical and mental life-style

IMPORTANT SAFETY INFORMATION

If you are in any doubt about your health or physical ability to exercise, you should consult a doctor before commencing any physical training program. If you are pregnant, if your health status has recently changed, if you have not exercised for the last six months, or if you have had a recent illness or injury, please consult your doctor.

It takes time to increase your overall level of fitness. Training too hard or too fast is a common cause of exercise and sports-related injuries. Suggestions include:

- See your doctor for a full medical check-up before embarking on any new fitness program.

- Warm up thoroughly by performing slow, sustained stretches and going through the motions of your sport or activity.

- Use proper form and technique while exercising.

- Wear proper attire.

- Stay hydrated.

- Always cool down after exercise with plenty of slow stretching.

See your doctor for regular medical check-ups.

INTRODUCTION

1

Firefighting is a hazardous, sometime life-threatening occupation. Many professional firefighters are usually selected for their excellent physical fitness, firefighting experience, and likelihood of success with professional training. Because of the rigorous demands placed on them, most have to demonstrate above-average physical stamina and strength upon entry into the profession (Bogucki & Rabinowitz, 2004). However, Bauer (2011) suggested that many firefighters are no fitter than the average sedentary individual. In fact, many firefighters are found to be overweight and have high levels of cholesterol, which lead to cardiac disease. During normal duty hours, most firefighters face long periods of down time when they get little or no exercise, but when an emergency occurs, sudden, intense energy is needed to fight a fire. This increase of energy can place those in poor health in grave danger but can also create concern for public safety (Kales, Soteriades, Christophi, and Christiani, 2007).

It has been well documented that the number-one killer of firefighters is heart disease. Intervention strategies within a comprehensive health and wellness program have helped to reduce these numbers over the years, but there is still an alarming rate of firefighters who suffer from heart attacks each year.

Researchers at Iowa State University discovered that 86 percent of volunteer firefighters did not know their blood lipid level and 47 percent did not know their blood pressure. Within the US alone, over one million people will suffer a heart attack within the next year and it does not just affect the elderly. We are now seeing individuals as young as twenty-one suffer from heart disease.

Sleep plays an important role in helping our bodies recover from stress, illness, and fatigue. If we do not get quality sleep, our resting metabolic rate will decrease, causing weight gain. A firefighter's "internal biological clock" is often disrupted throughout a shift, affecting the body's ability to regulate the sleep-wake system. Researchers at the Brigham and Women's Hospital showed that prolonged sleep restriction with simultaneous circadian disruption decreased the individual's metabolic rate, thereby increasing over time the risk of diabetes.

The University of Chicago (1999) went even further and showed there is a direct link between sleeping and an increased risk of stroke, heart attack, and congestive heart failure. Their findings show how an individual who sleeps more than eight hours and less than six has a significantly higher chance of chest pain or angina and coronary heart disease. Therefore it is important to control the duration of restful sleep in a completely dark room to help reduce the chances of heart disease and other related illnesses.

Being overweight also is attributed to heart disease. Abdominal fat, also known as visceral fat, is generally associated with diabetes. However, there have been links to an increase of strokes through the hardening of the arteries. Increased visceral fat could lead to diabetes, which creates a change in blood vessels that reduce blood flow to the brain. Based on the findings at Iowa State University, 41 percent of volunteer firefighters were classified as obese, and 35 percent classified as overweight. Therefore it is recommended that a firefighter participate in physical activity and a proper nutrition program to reverse the side effects associated with belly fat.

Firefighters are often exposed to traumatic stress. According to researchers at the University of California—San Francisco (Cohen, 2012), these exposures over a lifetime or career will boost inflammation in the body, even if they do not lead to post-traumatic stress disorder. It was discovered that the greater the traumatic stress, the higher levels of inflammation within the body. Individuals with higher levels of inflammation within their body tend to have an increased risk of having a heart attack. Even if the firefighter adjusted to these traumatic events, the inflammation remained constant over a period of time. So the stress of the job can impact your health even if you don't have certain mental or physical symptoms. Intervention strategies to help combat stress, such as exercise, yoga, and other health-related activities, should be integrated at the start of a firefighter's career.

Firefighting itself is physical demanding and will eventually break the body down. According to a study performed at the Illinois Fire Service Institute (Fernhall,

2011), three hours of prolonged firefighting stiffens arteries and impairs heart function in young healthy male firefighters. The same is seen within heavy powerlifters and ultra marathon runners.

This could affect those firefighters who do not value the importance of fitness and therefore exhibit several of the risk factors for cardiovascular disease, including being overweight and having elevated blood pressure and/or cholesterol.

Finally your lungs; breathing in toxic fumes and particles during overhaul, exhaust pollution from the app bay, and exposures during most regular calls can adversely affect lung function. Lung function and obstructive airway diseases are strongly and independently associated with increased risk of heart failure. These results were not primarily confronted by just smokers, but also non-smokers.

Increased physical fitness can improve a firefighter's ability to perform specific job functions as well as offer resistance to cardiopulmonary conditions, and it is recommended that periodic testing be performed with individualized prescriptions for all active firefighters (Peate, 2002). The National Fire Protection Agency (NFPA) and the International Association of Firefighters (IAAF) recommend that all firefighters take part in some sort of physical fitness training to ensure that the physical requirements of fighting fire are addressed and to ensure public safety (Karter and Molis, 2006).

Preparing for a career in the fire service starts before entry into the academy. Recruits need to prepare themselves physically in order to withstand the strenuous workload and extreme working conditions in order to increase their success rate. The goal of a fire academy is to train firefighters, emergency medical technicians, and paramedics for professional response to the public needs. Recruits generally attend the academy for approximately three months (standard forty-hour work week) to improve their minds and bodies in fire science, safety, fire extinguishing systems, fire service hydraulics, vehicle extrication, physical conditioning, and more.

Physical training is an important component of the academy. All candidates must be in good physical condition before entrance into the academy. Those who are unable to perform typical firefighting tasks due to a lack of physical conditioning usually are not accepted into an academy. Although not all departments require an entrance physical, it is encouraged that recruits consult their doctor before starting any exercise program.

The content within this book are divided up to help individuals understand the risks involved with fire suppression as well as to prepare them for a career and a career in the fire service.

Chapter 2: Overview of the Fire Service looks at the current injuries, illness, deaths, and other health concerns that are related to the fire service.

Chapter 3: Major Fire Services Wellness Initiatives explains how the fire service is taking a proactive approach in regards to health and wellness within fire suppression. It examines current initiatives that are being incorporated to protect the firefighter's health.

Chapter 4: Importance of Health and Wellness in the Fire Service explains the science behind the health concerns related to firefighters. It will provide the recruit with a good understanding of the health risks involved with fire suppression and motivate the recruit to maintain a healthy lifestyle upon graduation and throughout their career.

Chapters 5 and 6: What Is Physical Fitness? And **How to Develop and Maintain Physical Fitness** explains how a recruit can develop their overall physical fitness before entrance into an academy. It covers the different physiological components, such as cardiovascular, resistance training, and flexibility.

Chapter 7: Nutrition Information explains the concepts of basic nutrition and hydration and how they will help increase physical conditioning as well as create a healthier lifestyle.

This manual ends with appendices that provide examples of cardiovascular training programs, resistance training programs, training logs, and flexibility programs.

2

OVERVIEW OF THE FIRE SERVICE

There are 1,148,100 firefighters in the US. Of those, 335,950 (29 percent) are career firefighters and 812,150 (72 percent) are volunteers. Most career firefighters (71 percent) are working in communities that protect twenty-five thousand people or more. Volunteer firefighters (95 percent) are in departments that protect less than twenty-five thousand people, with more than half located in small, rural departments that protect fewer than twenty-five hundred people. In 2009, it was estimated that there were 30,165 fire departments in the US. Of these, 2,457 are all career, 1,752 are mostly career, 5,099 are mostly volunteer, and 20,857 are all volunteer. In the US, 44 percent of fire departments provide emergency medical services (EMS), 15 percent provide EMS service and advanced life support, while 41 percent of departments provide no EMS support. Fire department types did vary considerably by population.

While fighting structure fires remains a core function of fire departments, several other areas are also incorporated. Firefighters must respond to medical emergencies, hazardous materials, motor vehicle accidents, and rescue situations. In 2009, medical aid accounted for 65 percent of all fire department calls, whereas 5 percent were attributed to actual fires. All these activities must be performed while wearing heavy fire-retardant clothing, helmet, self-contained breathing apparatus (SCBA), and other protective gear that may weigh in excess of fifty pounds. These occupational hazards create an unstable environment that creates high rates of work-related illnesses, injuries, or mortality. Because of increased risks in musculoskeletal injuries and cardiac complications, most fire departments are establishing physical conditioning programs.

CONCERNS IN THE FIRE SERVICE

In 2009, 78,150 firefighting injuries occurred; this is a decrease of 1.9 percent from a year before. A total of 32,205 (41 percent) of all firefighting injuries occurred during fire-ground operations, which has been the lowest since 1981. Another 17,590 (22 percent) occurred during other on-duty activities, while 15,455 (20 percent) occurred at non-fire emergency incidents. The leading type of injury received during fire ground operations was strain, sprain, or muscular pain (48.2 percent), followed by wound, cut, bleeding, bruise (13.2 percent), and smoke or gas inhalation (8 percent). The leading causes of fire-ground injuries were overexertion, strain (25.2 percent) and falls, slips, or jumps (22.7 percent). For non-fire injuries, strains, sprains, and muscular pain accounted for 58.9 percent. The NFPA estimates that there were 11,900 cases of exposure to infectious diseases and twenty-three thousand exposures to hazardous conditions. An estimated 15,150 (19.4 percent) of all firefighters' injuries resulted in lost time in 2009.

It is recommend that a health and wellness program be established within fire departments as well as the application of existing technology to help reduce levels of injury and bring about corresponding reductions that are recommended by NFPA 1583 (2008).

The next section provides some insight into some of the leading risk factors that are associated with firefighting.

CARDIOVASCULAR:

In 2009, ninety firefighters died while on duty, which was the lowest total since 1993, yet thirty-nine of those deaths were attributed to coronary heart disease (CAD). Of those, a total of thirty-six deaths were of career firefighters, forty-seven of volunteers, and seven part- or full-time members of wildland agencies. Based on the latest report by the US Fire Administration (FEMA, 2010), coronary heart disease is the leading cause of death among firefighters.

In one study performed by the *New England Journal of Medicine* (Kales, 2007), 32 percent of all deaths were related to coronary heart disease. Of those deaths, 13.4 percent were responding to an alarm, 17.4 percent were returning from an alarm, 12.5 percent were engaged in physical training, 9.4 percent were responding to a non-emergency, and 15.4 percent were performing a non-emergency. Occurrence of a heart attack is 12.1 to 136 times more likely to happen during fire suppression, 2.8 to 14.1 more likely to happen during an alarm response, 2.2 to 10.5 as high during an alarm response, and 2.9 to 6.6 times as high during physical training.

Because these findings are so crucial to the lives of firefighters, it is imperative that they establish healthy habits before entering into an academy and therefore reduce the risk of having coronary artery disease throughout their career.

STRAINS AND SPRAINS:

Injuries are costing the fire service millions of dollars annually. Firefighters are not representative of the typical population. The job demands are similar to those of an elite athlete. Studies have shown that exertion and cardiovascular levels can reach extremely high levels quickly and for long periods of time. In one study performed by the University of Portsmouth (Eglin, 2007), it was found that a firefighter should have an aerobic capacity (VO$_2$ max) of **42 ml·kg$^-$·min^{-1}** to meet the physical demands brought on by fire suppression. It is also recommended that fire recruits have a VO$_2$ max of **45 ml·kg^{-1}·min^{-1} upon entry into an academy**. Another area to factor in is the impact and stress the joints take as a result of carrying and wearing more than fifty pounds of personal protective equipment (PPE) and gear—and with no time to warm up or stretch, it is not surprising that chronic and recurring injuries are far too prevalent. Research conducted by York University (Ontario) about the physical demands of firefighting stated that a firefighter's applications of strength and endurance were lifting and carrying objects (up to eighty pounds), pulling objects (up to 135 pounds), and working with objects in front of the body (up to 125 pounds). The cost estimated for all firefighter injuries is between $5 to 8 billion overall.

In 2009, back injuries were the most common injury, followed by shoulder and knee injury. In the last two years, knee injuries will most likely result in costs greater than ten thousand dollars than back and shoulder injuries. According to the International Association of Firefighters (IAFF)—Firefighter Death and Injury Survey (2000), nearly one in five firefighters is injured in the line of duty. It was also concluded that the rate of injury was three times higher in the fire industry than in the private sector.

Based on the NFPA—Firefighter Injuries (2010), the major types of injuries that occur during fire-ground operations are as follows:

· Strain, sprain, muscular pain (48.2 percent)

· Wound, cut, bleeding (13.2 percent)

· Burns (7.1 percent)

· Thermal stress (frostbite, heat exhaustion) [5.8 percent]

· Smoke or gas inhalation (6.2 percent)

Strain, sprains, and muscular pain accounted for 61.4 percent during non-fire ground operations.

Some of the contributing factors for these injuries are rapid response requirement with no time for preparation, restrictive PPE, visual restriction, functional movement (especially with SCBA), increased work effort, significant lifting, movement of heavy objects, and awkward positions without adequate core body support.

Because of the increased risks in musculoskeletal injuries and cardiac complications, many fire departments are establishing health and wellness programs. Increasing firefighters' physical fitness will aid them in performing such tasks as pulling hoses, carrying equipment up and down ladders and stairs, forced entry into structures, and carrying victims to safety (Findley, Brown, Whitehurst, Gilbert, and Apold, 2002).

SLEEP:

Proper nutrition, exercise, and adequate sleep are the foundations for a healthy lifestyle. Because of the variety of shift schedules many firefighters work, many do not get the required six to ten hours of sleep to function properly. Many firefighters claim that sleep disturbances were considered an important part of increased stress levels.

Sleep is an active state affecting both physical and mental well-being. The average adult needs seven to eight hours of sleep per night, but individual needs vary and range from five to ten hours a night.

Sleep debt is sleep loss that accumulates from one night to the next. Acute sleep deprivation is less than four to six hours of sleep in a twenty-four-hour period. Even a modest loss of sleep may produce a serious sleep debt when sustained over several consecutive nights. Inadequate sleep results in reduced attention, concentration, and memory; fatigue; higher stress levels; and personality changes, particularly loss of humor or increased ill temper. Other effects include shortened temper, lower motivation, slower reflexes, and higher error rates. The only way to reduce sleep debt is to get the amount of sleep your body needs.

Workers in industries that have shifts, such as firefighting, are more prone to heart attacks, ulcers, depression, and serious sleep disorders than normal day workers. They are three to four times more likely to have sleep apnea than the normal population.

Based on the study conducted by Elliot and Kuehl (2007), chronic sleep deprivation and long work hours are linked to a general increase in health complaints, obesity, obstructive sleep apnea, and possible heightened risk for cardiovascular disease.

IMPORTANT FACTS:

- Firefighter should have an aerobic capacity (VO_2 max) of **$42\,ml\cdot kg^{-1}\cdot min^{-1}$.**

- Fire recruits have a VO_2 max of **$45\ ml\cdot kg^{-1}\cdot min^{-1}$ upon entry into an academy.**

- Firefighters should be able to carry objects (up to eighty pounds), pull objects (up to 135 pounds), and work with objects in front of the body (up to 125 pounds).

- Most injuries for career firefighters occur between the ages of thirty and thirty-nine.

- Most injuries for volunteer firefighters occur between the ages of twenty and twenty-nine.

- The leading cause of death among firefighters is coronary heart disease.

- In 2009, thirty-nine firefighter deaths were contributed to coronary heart disease (CAD).

- Back injuries were the most common injury, followed by shoulder and knee injury.

- **Sleep deprivation**: a sufficient lack of restorative sleep over a _cumulative period_ so as to cause physical or psychiatric symptoms and affect routine performances of tasks

- **Sleep apnea**: a breathing disorder characterized by brief interruptions of breathing during sleep

3

OVERVIEW OF MAJOR FIRE SERVICES WELLNESS INITIATIVES

Health and wellness are a top priority in the fire service. Equipment such as trucks, engines, hoses, and other apparatus can be fixed or replaced, but the firefighter cannot. Many resources go into the well-being of a firefighter and many departments feel it is their responsibility to provide and protect their employees. According to the NFPA, in 2010 the percentage of California fire departments with no health and wellness program was 41 percent, compared to 64 percent in 2005 and 61percent in 2001. By establishing a successful wellness program, many departments often increase the overall health of its members, as well as increase public safety.

It has been researched in numerous studies that firefighters are an especially high-risk group for musculoskeletal injuries and other work-related health problems. In one study performed by the Oregon Health and Science University, it was found that most fire agencies focus more on maintenance of their apparatus but repair their firefighters when injured (Table 2).

	Fire Apparatus	Firefighter
Maintenance	70%	3%
Repair	30%	97%
TOTAL	100%	100%

Table 2: COST OF MAINTENANCE AND REPAIR (Percent of Budget)
Source: Kuehl (Jan. 2005) Phlame Study

NFPA STANDARDS

In August of 2000, the NFPA released *NFPA 1583: Standard on Health-Related Fitness Programs for Firefighters.* As stated by the NFPA, "The intent of this document is to provide the minimum requirement of the development, implementation, and management for a health-related fitness program (HRFP). It is not intended to establish physical performance criteria, and to be non-punitive."

To further develop a department's health and wellness program and complement the NFPA 1583, the NFPA also created the *NFPA 1582—Comprehensive Occupational Medical Program for Fire Departments*. The intent of this standard is to provide the following:

- A national consensus standard on entry requirements for firefighters

- A national consensus standard on medical guidance for managing current fire members

- A consistent guide for development and implementation of a comprehensive occupational medicine program for fire departments

- The function of the fire department physician (as well as defining it)

IAFF/IAFC FIRE SERVICE JOINT LABOR WELLNESS FITNESS INITIATIVES (WFI)

The IAFF/IAFC–WFI established *"The 10 Cities Initiative,"* which utilizes some of North America's finest fire departments to improve the health and wellness of fire department personnel.

Based on the Kuehle-Redmond study (Jan. 2005), the ten departments within the WFI program had a savings of $1,336,535 per year compared to fire departments that did not implement a health and wellness program. This program is based on the premise that the program in non-punitive and confidential. For any program to succeed, it is recommended they adopt these same conditions.

4

IMPORTANCE OF HEALTH AND WELLNESS IN THE FIRE SERVICE

Professional firefighters are generally selected on the basis of their excellent physical fitness, firefighting experience, and likelihood of success with professional training. Cardio respiratory fitness, muscular strength, muscular endurance, flexibility, and a healthy body composition are important not only for occupational requirements but also for the safety of the firefighters, co-workers, and the general public. But previous studies have shown that there is a decrease in physical performance in both the general population and firefighters as they increase in age. Cardiac risk factors can increase with age, and because of the increased occupational stressors involved with firefighting, many fire departments are seeking methods to prevent any coronary risk factors.

The study performed by Davis, Jankovitz, and Rein (2002) observed that firefighters had higher physical fitness levels compared to the general population at any given age. Yet there was a dramatic reduction in physical fitness across the career span for a firefighter. Increased blood cholesterol, body fat mass, and blood pressure occurred with age. Other cardiac risk factors are a cause for concern among firefighters, especially with the increased stressors involved with the occupation. This shows the importance of a health and wellness program within a fire department.

A comprehensive training program includes the following components:

- Regular fitness screenings and tiered medical assessments

- Aerobic output

- Anaerobic output

- Resistance training

- Flexibility

- Hydration

- Nutrition

- Rehabilitation

When a program combines all of these components, the firefighters may pay more attention to their personal health and wellness, which will improve public safety.

REGULAR FITNESS SCREENINGS AND MEDICAL ASSESSMENTS

Regular screening and medical assessments are an important foundation for a successful, comprehensive health and wellness program. NFPA 1582 provides a set of guidelines for medical testing and screening, which simplifies the development of this component. All fitness screenings and medical assessments should be non-punitive yet mandatory. The purpose of these assessments is to perform health screening, not primary care.

FITNESS SCREENING

Prior to participation in any fitness program, firefighters should be effectively screened in accordance with the American College of Sports Medicine (ACSM) guidelines. These guidelines will classify individuals as low, moderate, or high risk for participation in any fitness program that is in use. Individuals classified as high risk should be referred to a high-risk intervention program, closely supervised by medical personnel.

TIERED MEDICAL EXAMINATION

NFPA 1582 recommends an annual medical examination for firefighters over forty years of age, at least every two years for those between ages thirty and thirty-nine, and at least every three years for those ages twenty-nine and under. Examinations should be standardized for all members. The overall tiered medical program is designed to assess the five most common health issues faced by our firefighters: obesity, hypertension, lung disease, cardiac wellness, and diabetes. The objective of the program would be to identify and render assistance to members who need intervention. There would be no intention of removal from duty unless a medical condition warrants. Removal to alternate duty is non-punitive and intended for medical rehabilitation, and assistance is focused to get the member back to lower tiers as quickly as possible. Below is an example (Table 4) of a tired medical program used by the Phoenix Fire Department.

Health Standards	Tier 4	Tier 3	Tier 2	Tier 1
Body Fat %	>30% Male	25-30% M	20-24% M	<20% M
	>34% Female	30-34% F	24-29% F	<24% F
Blood Pressure	>160/110	>150/100	>140/90	<135/85
FEV¹ / FVC%	<59%	<65%	<75%	>75%
METS	< 12.0	12.0-12.9	13.0-13.9	>14.0
Blood Sugar HbA¹	>300	200-299	100-199	65-99
	8.0	>7.5	6.5-7.4	<6.5

Table 4: PHOENIX FIRE DEPARTMENT TIERED MEDICAL PROGRAM

HEALTH RISKS:

CARDIOVASCULAR DISEASE

Cardiac-related deaths are the leading cause of mortality among firefighters. It is also the most common cause of death from disease in the US. One out of every three men in the US will die from heart disease. Each year, 1.5 million heart attacks occur in the United States, and 25 percent of them end fatally.

There are many types of heart disease, including diseases of the heart valves, the heart muscle, and the arteries that take blood to the heart muscle. The most common heart disease is coronary heart disease, which is a narrowing of the arteries that supply the heart with blood.

There are some excellent screening measures that could help us predict heart disease before it happens. The most common measures are: blood pressure (BP) monitoring, lipid testing, C-reactive protein (CRP), electrocardiogram (ECG), and stress ECG/exercise stress test.

Another excellent screening tool is the measuring of metabolic equivalent rates (METS) on cardiac stress testing. While this is not as good as a full diagnostic testing (such as measuring for VO_2 max) or doing stress echocardiography, stress ECGs still provide reliable, reproducible results that effectively measure cardiac tone.

The goals of cardiac health should be to identify the individuals who are showing decreased cardiac tone, ensure there are no underlying medical reasons, and, if so, provide the appropriate medical therapy.

According to a study performed at the Illinois Fire Service Institute (2011), three hours of prolonged firefighting stiffens arteries and impairs heart function in young healthy male firefighters.

The same things occur in athletes who perform maximal aerobic or heavy resistance exercises. For young athletes (under thirty-five), sudden cardiac death is caused mainly by inherited structural and functional abnormalities, while in the over-thirty-fives it can be attributed primarily to coronary artery disease. **Both of these conditions can be diagnosed through screening.**

Usually a stiff artery is associated with an increase in inflammation and blood pressure. Each year the leading cause of death for firefighters is heart attacks, and many times when we go to the doctor we get our cholesterol checked but neglect our C-reactive protein.

C-reactive protein is a marker of the intensity of early inflammation in myocardial infarction, which predicts long-term mortality and heart failure. Studies have shown that it could be a better predictor because it provides analytical information beyond that provided by conventional risk factors and the degree of left ventricular systolic dysfunction (it has also been linked to Alzheimer's disease and dementia).

What we do know from this study is that artery stiffness and cardiac fatigues did occur. It has been shown that exercise-induced cardiac fatigue (or a reduction of cardiac function) occurs following prolonged strenuous exercise. In a study carried out in the 1960s, athletes were found to exhibit a significant decrease in stroke volume (the amount of blood pumped out by the heart in a single beat) following a bout of prolonged exercise. This established a possible link between exhaustive exercise and the potential for a decrease in cardiac function. Skeletal muscle fatigues after a period of extended exercise and the heart is a muscle, but it cannot rest. It has to supply the body with blood, and therefore never gets to take a break.

Cardiac fatigue has been demonstrated in healthy subjects following a twenty-kilometer run and a sixty-minute cycle ride. It is possible that cardiac fatigue may affect firefighters as well as the elite athletes taking part in ultra-endurance events. Athletes spend months preparing for their event, whereas many firefighters do not value the important of fitness and therefore exhibit several of the risk factors for cardiovascular disease, including being overweight and having elevated blood pressure and/or cholesterol. Now include the actual physical and psychological stressors involved with the job—heat stress exacerbated by heavy gear that doesn't allow the body to cool, acute periods of aerobic and resistance exercise, and activation of the "fight or flight" response of the sympathetic nervous system—and you are asking for trouble.

It is worth noting that there is no evidence to support the existence of cardiac fatigue following periods of intense ***brief*** exercise. In studies of relatively short periods of endurance exercise (fifty to one hundred fifty minutes), cardiac fatigue has not always been observed. As a result, it has been suggested that exercise duration may be an important factor in determining the onset of cardiac fatigue, although the existence of a serious 'threshold' has not been established. Other factors, such as temperature and humidity, altitude, hydration status, gender, and age, may also be significant, and differences in these variables may account for some of the conflicting findings in the current literature.

Overall, a regular endurance training program will, in fact, ultimately benefit the heart and reduce the risk of major heart disease in the long term. However, it is important to remind people embarking on intensive training programs (especially sedentary firefighters) that it is advisable to undergo a full cardiovascular screening and to take a sensible approach toward an exercise program.

Based on the results of the Illinois Fire Service Institute study the firefighter's endothelial function—blood flow as controlled by the inner lining of blood vessels—improved after the firefighting exercise. This is generally seen in athletes who perform heavy resistance exercises. This can be attributed to the fact that firefighters do a lot of resistance-type exercise when they're fighting a fire: handling heavy equipment, doing forcible entry, and other tasks that increase blood flow in their arms, which is where endothelial function was measured. Endothelial dysfunction is emerging as a significant complication for a person battling type-1 diabetes.

QUICK TIPS

- One recent study performed at the Institute of Health Science and Applied Physiology (2007) showed that cardio after weight lifting seemed to cure the arterial stiffness issue. T**o help combat arterial stiffness, perform aerobic training after resistance training**.

- Not all heavy resistance training [*"Cardiovascular responses to short-term Olympic style weight-training in young men"* (1983)] found that their systolic actually decreased. Another similar study found that weight training **decreased diastolic blood pressure, raised HDL, lowered cholesterol, and decreased insulin levels**, all big risk factors for heart disease.

- Cardiac fatigue has not always been seen in short periods of endurance exercise (fifty to one hundred fifty minutes), so use a sensible approach to exercise.

C-REACTIVE PROTEIN

o   You are at low risk of developing cardiovascular disease if your hs-CRP level is lower than 1.0mg/L.

o   You are at average risk of developing cardiovascular disease if your levels are between 1.0 and 3.0 mg/L.

o   You are at high risk for cardiovascular disease if your hs-CRP level is higher than 3.0 mg/L.

HYPERTENSION

Hypertension is still the leading risk factor for heart disease and stroke. Elevated blood pressures have both acute and chronic health concerns, which usually improve with exercise and diet. Medication is still the most effective means for control.

Your chance of developing cardiovascular disease (heart attacks and strokes) increases when your systolic blood pressure (SBP) is at or above 140 mm Hg or the diastolic blood pressure (DPB) reaches or exceeds 90 mm Hg. Exercise reduces your chance of having high blood pressure by 50 percent, and if you already have hypertension, regular physical fitness activity can take about 10 mm Hg off your systolic and diastolic pressure. If you already take several medications, exercise can reduce the number of medications you need for treatment.

Our blood cholesterol level relates to our risk of coronary artery disease. The higher our low-density lipoprotein (LDL) or "bad" cholesterol, the more likely those fatty deposits build up on the walls of our arteries, slowly squeezing off the blood supply. By limiting the amount of saturated fat you consume, you can reduce your total and LDL cholesterol. High-density lipoprotein (HDL) is our "good" cholesterol. The HDL helps remove the fatty build-up from our arteries and carries harmful cholesterol back to the liver for destruction. The higher our HDL, the more protection we have from heart and blood vessel disease. When our HDL cholesterol drops below 35 mg/dL, our risk for coronary heart disease increases. One can increase their HDL through exercise, reducing their body fat, and a healthier diet.

The goals for hypertension would be to work with the member to effect health changes, provide an immediate referral to their primary care provider, address any underlying health issues, and monitor their progress.

OBESITY

Obesity is now the second leading cause of mortality in the US. Body fat percentage (BF%) is a leading precursor for adult onset diabetes, hypertension, and heart disease. More than half Americans are overweight or obese, based on the current definitions.

High blood sugar or diabetes mellitus is a major risk for coronary heart disease and stroke. One of the most severe consequences of diabetes is that it silently accelerates the blood-vessel-narrowing processes and intensifies the harm of other cardiac risk factors. Children and young adults usually have type-1 diabetes or insulin-dependent diabetes mellitus. This is most often caused by the body's overactive immune system, destroying the insulin-producing cells of the pancreas. Type-2 diabetes is also known as adult onset or non-insulin diabetes mellitus. This type of diabetes has a generic component and is most often related to not exercising and being overweight. Exercise can help eliminate this form of diabetes entirely and/or reduce the need for blood-sugar-lowering medication.

THE METABOLIC SYNDROME

If an individual has at least three of the five below, they probably have the metabolic syndrome or insulin resistance, which increases your risk of heart disease, diabetes, and dementia. The treatment is regular exercise and weight loss.

Abdominal Obesity

High Blood Triglyceride Levels

Low HDL Cholesterol Levels

Elevated Blood Pressure (Greater than 130/85)

Elevated Fasting Blood Sugar (Greater than 100)

Body fat goals would be to work with the member to effect health changes, identify any reasons for obesity, address the underlying health issues, provide any assistance with a dietician and fitness trainer, and monitor their progress.

PULMONARY DISEASE

Lung function is a big concern among firefighters. Members who are subjected to significant hazardous chemical exposures have a great risk of lung disease. There is also an epidemic of asthma and other reactive airway diseases in the country, and this could be reflected in our fire departments.

There is a big controversy right now in firefighting medicine on how to handle members with asthma, as well as acceptability of candidates with a history of asthma.

Asthma can kill, and has been associated with at least two member fatalities in FDNY.

In most cases with asthma, we do not want just to see members with good lungs reserved under normal circumstances, but we also want to see a history of good control of the disease. Using pulmonary function test results is just a guide in evaluating asthma. By measuring the percentage of air exhaled in the first second is a great indicator of obstructive lung disease (FEV1/FVC).

Another important fact that is not listed are that those members whose FVC (total amount of air exhaled) is less than 80 percent also have an indication of a significant health issue that needs to be individually addressed.

It is very challenging dealing with members with pulmonary diseases. Each case must be dealt with individually. It must deal with the underlying lung function and help maximize that function. Then they must truly assess the member's ability to perform functions safely without further impacting on the disease.

CANCER

Cancer is a group of many related diseases. All cancers share out-of-control cell growth and spread abnormal cells. Cancer cells accumulate and form tumors that may compress, invade, and destroy normal tissue. If cells break away from a tumor, they can travel through the bloodstream or the lymph system to other areas of the body. The spread of a tumor to a new site is called a metastasis. Cancer is classified by the part of the body in which it began and by its appearance under a microscope. Different cancers vary in their cell type, rates of growth, patterns of spread, and responses to different types of treatment. That is one of the reasons that people with cancer need treatment that is aimed at the specific problem.

Different cancers have different risk factors. A risk factor is anything that increases a person's chance of developing a disease, such as a cancer. However, they do not explain everything about why a person develops an illness.

The best known cancer risk factor is cigarette smoking. The American Cancer Society estimates that about 175,000 cancer deaths per year are caused by tobacco use. An even bigger adverse effect of smoking is heart disease, which is greatly accelerated by smoking. Greater consumption of vegetables, fruits, or both together has also been associated with a lower risk of lung cancer. The major risk factor for lung cancer is tobacco, but diet also affects risk.

A healthy diet and regular exercise can promote health and reduce your cancer risk. Evidence suggests that about one-third of the 500,000 cancer deaths that occur in the United States each year are due to dietary factors. Cancer risk can be reduced by a diet high in plant foods (fruits and vegetables), limited in meat, dairy, and other high-saturated-fat foods, and balanced in calories and physical activity. These dietary recommendations are also the same as those that help prevent coronary heart disease, diabetes, and other lifestyle-related chronic conditions.

SEVEN EARLY WARNINGS OF CANCER

Any persistent change in bowel or bladder function

Any sore that does not heel

Unusual bleeding or discharge (for example, coughing up blood, abnormal vaginal bleeding or discharge, or blood in the stool)

A thickening or lump in the breast or elsewhere

Persistent indigestion or difficulty swallowing

Recent change in the size or color of a wart or mole

A nagging cough or hoarseness lasting more than two weeks

JOINT AND BACK PROBLEMS

One in seven Americans has arthritis. The most common type is osteoarthritis (OA), which is also called degenerative joint disease (DJD) or "wear-and-tear" arthritis. It primarily affects older adults. The older you are, the more likely you are to have DJD.

Arthritis means joint inflammation, and the joints usually affected by OA are in your hands and the weight-bearing joints in your legs. OA of the hands and hips tends to run in families. Being overweight, diabetic, or having poor physical health will increase your chances of having arthritis.

Exercise can help joints damaged from arthritis. It does not damage joints. In fact, even if you already have arthritis, your joints benefit from regular physical activity. Joint movement helps keep healthy cartilage by stimulating it to take up nutrients and dispose of waste products. In addition, exercise strengthens muscles, so that they can better support our joints.

TIPS FOR EXERCISING WITH OSTEOARTHRITIS

Choose exercises that minimize joint stress and strengthen muscles around arthritic joints.

Seek advice about specific exercises to stabilize joints and correct biomechanical problems.

Ask whether a brace, elastic wrap, or taping would be helpful.

After discussing it with your physician, you may consider taking aspirin or a nonsteroidal anti-inflammatory drug (NSAID) before exercising and icing a joint immediately after your workout.

Warm up your muscles and joints before exercise and use gentle stretches to increase joint flexibility.

Eighty percent of us will have back pain sometime in our lives. Back pain is very common and usually not due to serious disease. Firefighters typically have back pain that is caused from overuse, straining, or improper body mechanics.

Most back pain will improve in a week, and 90 percent by three months after its onset. Most people with back pain do not have any damage in their spine. In fact, it is very difficult to damage your spine. Many also do not have a herniated disk or pinched nerve. It may feel as if all you can do is lie in bed with an ice pack, but do not stay there too long. Studies have shown that your back pain improves just as fast when you are up and moving around.

Once you are pain-free, you can begin a regular exercise routine to strengthen the spine's supporting muscles. Both increasing your back muscles and increasing your overall endurance can help keep your backache from coming back.

Piriformis syndrome is a common cause for "pain in the butt." The piriformis muscle is deep within your glute. If the muscle is overworked, it can go into spasm. This causes pain in the center of your gluteal. Because the muscle pinches your sciatic nerve, pain can shoot down the back of your leg. Self-myofascial release, icing the muscle and specific stretches will help relax the muscle and remedy the problem.

Table 5 has more information to protect your back.

TABLE 5: BODY MECHANICS TO DECREASE BACK PAIN

- Avoid loading the spine.
- Keep the load closer to your body.
- Utilize the golfer's lift to minimize low back motion and loads on the low back.
- Push forces directed through the low back minimize the moment and spine load. For example: when pushing a vacuum, you want to push it while in front of the body (in front of belly button), not on the side, which creates large twisting and vectors on the spine.
- There is NO IDEAL SITTING POSTURE! If you are sitting for prolonged periods of time, change your sitting posture to allow more variable movement.
- If you sit for long periods of time, GET UP! A rest break must consist of the opposite activity to reduce the imposed stress. Stand normal for ten to twenty seconds, then reach for the ceiling, stretch, and push the hands upward then inhale deeply and slowly.
- Perform back exercises during the midday (most ideal) but NEVER IN THE MORNING.
- Sit in a taller chair with angled seat pads. This will help extend the hips and lumbar spine.
- AVOID FLEXION OF THE SPINE: The most successful programs appear to emphasize trunk stabilization through exercise with a neutral spine while stressing mobility at the hips and knees.
- WALKING IS GREAT, but fast walking with the arms swinging results in lower oscillating spine load. When tolerable, aerobic exercise, particularly fast walking, appears to enhance the effects of back-specific exercises, so try to get some in.
- Train to breathe feely while maintaining the stabilizing contractions within the core.
- Low back exercises appear to be most beneficial when performed daily and in the midday (if possible).
- DO NOT PERFORM FULL RANGE SPINE MOTIN UNDER LOAD one to two hours after getting out of bed.
- NO MORE than eight hours in bed. Prolonged lying down will only make things worse.

SHOULDER PAIN

It is well documented that firefighting is a physically demanding job and throughout their career firefighters will deal with some type of injury (i.e., low back, knee, shoulder). Shoulder problems are starting to become more apparent with firefighters due to a number of factors, such as a reduction in thoracic spine mobility, rotator cuff endurance, and scapula stability. These attributes develop over time because of the physical demands required during normal fire-ground operations. If we include poor exercise selection and technique within their fitness program, we will only begin to see an increase of shoulder injuries.

Many new types of training modalities are being exposed to the fire service, everything from high-intensity training to multi-planar, metabolic conditioning are being implemented so firefighters may improve on their fitness. Still one-third of all injuries in the fire service resulted in physical exercise activities (Poplin, 2011). Exercise like push-ups and pull-ups are very common within these types of modalities due to the simplicity and effectiveness, yet performed incorrectly with repetitive motion will eventually cause pain or discomfort within the shoulder.

The shoulder is a unit composed of the shoulder joint and shoulder girdle that requires a great amount of dynamic stability. The glenohumeral joint is a mobile system that is mostly controlled by the deltoid and the rotator cuff. The scapula is the anchor for the rotator cuff and creates stability within the joint. The main priority when using the shoulder is to have glenohumeral and scapula rhythm. When there is a muscular imbalance between them along with high repetition and high intensity exercises, injuries will occur.

The rotator cuffs (RTC) primary job is to stabilize or center the humeral head within the socket when the arm is moving. When it no longer works properly, the deltoid will overpower it and force the humeral head to hit the ceiling of the joint socket, creating an impingement (which leads to a tear). It is recommended that you limit or eliminate deltoid side raises and shoulder fly work if you currently have shoulder pain—you're only going to make things worse. Remember the RTC works as a whole; every time you raise your arm all four muscles work, and it has a low load threshold, so if you use too much weight you will injure it. When a tear occurs the injured firefighters will not be able to stabilize their shoulder, forcing their scapula up, creating a shrug motion. Most RTC injuries do not just happen; it is generally a progressive pathology that goes from irritation to inflammation to fraying to tearing.

Exercise such as kipping pull-ups, overhead press, or handstand push-ups should not be recommended for firefighters dealing with shoulder pain. Kipping pull-ups are a method of jerking and swinging your way through a pull-up versus using the actual strength and power of your muscles to get your chin over the bar. It requires strength and stability within the shoulder girdle, and can be seriously exhausting to the muscles, joints, and connective tissue. Common injuries that have occurred from kipping pull-ups (high-repetitive/high-intensity movements) are superior labrum from anterior to posterior tears (SLAP) and rotator cuff problems. SLAP tears occur within your labrum when it is subject to sudden stress, such as kicking out of the bottom of a pull-up. Pain will generally occur when you move your arm overhead (i.e., pulling ceiling), or throw (i.e., pulling hose).

Age and poor posture are two other contributing factors to shoulder pain. One-third of all firefighter injuries occur between the ages of thirty ti thirty-nine. This is significant in the prevention of injuries because during this time period most males begin to lose their flexibility, see a reduction in aerobic capacity, and gain weight. Over time firefighters will also develop poor posture that can be attributed to the job. It is not uncommon to see a firefighter with their scapula protracted and anterior tilted due to their SCBA. This position will decrease strength in the serratus and low traps and create tightness in the pectoral minor and upper traps.

Some of the more common injuries in the fire service are either related to pain in the acromioclavicular (AC) or glenohumeral joint. To help assess the shoulder, raise your arm above your head. If the pain is painful at the top, it will probably be an AC joint problem (impingement); if this occurs while lifting your arm but goes away when you reach the top, it will probably be a glenohumeral joint (rotator cuff) problem. Always refer to your medical professional for further evaluation.

Most firefighter will suffer from external impingement because of the constant overhead work found in firefighting. The pain is general, caused by the following:

direct pressure on the AC joint

horizontal adduction (pull your arm across your chest) overhead motion

horizontal pressing (i.e., bench press, push-up)

periods of inactivity

internal rotation

If external impingement is the issue, the firefighters need to modify their exercise programs accordingly:

Overhead activities

Modify/eliminate horizontal pressing (perform isometric hold push-ups with feet elevated or floor presses).

Incorporate more horizontal rows (TRX low row).

Incorporate more scapula stabilization exercises (heavy farmer's walk).

Soft tissue work and stretch the pectoral minor, teres minor, and lats

Increase thoracic spine mobility (quadruped external rotation).

Rotator cuff problems are also very common in the fire service. They range from minor to severe. Specific pathologies associated with RTC problems are internal impingement, RTC tensile overload, and partial or full thickness tears. Most RTC injuries occur because of:

high reps with high intensity

high velocity

repetition and fatigue (arm fatigue and injury patterns)

To help reduce the chances of a shoulder injury occurring, firefighters should focus on creating rotator cuff balance by utilizing a 2:1 ratio of posterior to anterior exercises. External rotation should be used more so that the low trap and serratus begin to work together when you raise your arm, increasing scapula stability so that it will anchor the rotator cuff, reducing any impingements, developing dynamic stability, and never working the rotator to failure.

SAMPLE PROGRAM

Soft Tissue:

Foam Roller: lats, pec minor, teres minor

Static Stretch: pectoral minor, lat, and neck flexors

Activation: isometric hold push-ups with rhythmic stabilization (have someone gently push your body side to side, front and back while you maintain control—you should really feel your RTC working); heavy farmer's walk

Scapula Stabilization: W exercise (hands by your side and externally rotate your hands out so your elbows go down, creating a W; you will feel it in your mid back), prone Y exercise

External Rotation: side-lying shoulder rotation (with a towel between your arm and torso)

5

WHAT IS PHYSICAL FITNESS?

Many firefighters entering the fire academy do not have sufficient aerobic capacity levels to fight fires. It is only after they enter the academy and receive the proper physical training do they meet the necessary physical requirements (Roberts, O'Dea, Boyce, and Mannix, 2002). Generally, most training focuses on cardiovascular endurance and muscular endurance, but this does not provide the best evaluation of the overall demands of firefighting (Rhea, Alavar, and Gray, 2004). High-intensity interval training and circuit weight training have been introduced into some training programs, and have shown to have a significant increase on physical performance in many cadets in the academy (Pipes, 1977). Therefore, it is very important that both an aerobic and anaerobic training program be part of the firefighter's exercise prescription.

High levels of anaerobic power have been significantly correlated to job-specific tasks (Rhea, Alavar, and Gray, 2004). Hose operation, structure ventilation, stair climbing, and rescue operations all require a high amount of anaerobic output. Anaerobic output means without oxygen. It relates to short-term high-energy production where the predominant fuels are produced without the necessity of oxygen. The goal for anaerobic testing is to measure short durations (forty- to ninety-second) exercise bouts. Assessment of anaerobic performance can provide fitness experts with valuable information about the firefighter's fitness status as well as allowing them to monitor improvement throughout their training.

There is no question that exercise is needed in the fire service. It is a great way to maintain a healthy weight, curb cravings, promote good blood sugar levels, keep your mind sharp, and support your entire cardiovascular system. What type of cardiovascular exercise has been the latest argument? Should they be performing low-moderate intensity workouts or high-intensity workouts? The real answer is to do it on a consistent basis. There's no question that as exercise and activity levels increase, cardiovascular risk decreases.

So many fitness professionals will debate the importance of one over the other, but realistically they are both valuable tools. Which is more important is not significant, but rather the goal of the firefighter is significant. One specific goal all firefighters have is their maximal oxygen uptake (peak VO_2). Based on the recommendations of the IAFF/IAFC Wellness Fitness Initiative, a firefighters should have a peak VO_2 of no less than **42 ml·kg^{-1}·min^{-1}** to meet the physical demands of the job. Those who have a peak VO_2 of **33.5 ml·kg^{-1}·min^{-1}** or less have been determined to be at risk because they can only perform specific firefighter tasks for a few minutes (Tierney, 2010).

Coronary heart disease is the leading cause of death within the fire service, and those with a low aerobic capacity increase their chances of having a myocardial infarction by 90 percent (Peak, 2002). So the overall goal should be to improve the firefighter's aerobic capacity to a safe and effective level.

Weight loss is another goal of many firefighters. High-intensity training will primarily focus on caloric quantity by promoting weight loss by exercising hard and maximizing total caloric expenditure. On the other side, a long, slow run will focus on caloric quality and what type of fuel is being burned. Diet is the best method for overall weight loss, but it also helps determine what type of energy to burn. The correct training stimulus can determine what type of fuel we use during exercise and rest (Melanson, 2009). High-intensity training will burn carbohydrates and create adaptations that will improve your glycolytic capabilities, while also improving your ability to tolerate lactate and to efficiently convert it back to usable form of energy. However, for endurance athletes, energy coming from fat (low-intensity) spares the glycogen and saves unwanted muscle breakdown, helping them finish the race.

Fire suppression does utilize both aerobic and anaerobic energy systems. Let's look at a typical structure fire: the first few minutes are sizing up the scene, pulling the hose, and preparing to ventilate. Once the command has been given, fire attack is established and eventually the fire is extinguished. A normal self-contained breathing apparatus (SCBA) will last about twenty minutes during this entire process followed by rehab. This scenario would be considered high-intensity. However, the job is not completed and there is still overhaul, cleaning, and other specific tasks required, which could be classified as low-intensity. Sometime during this scenario the firefighter will have a crossover point or ventilator threshold (VT). This is when the body switches its primary fuel from fat to carbohydrates. The goal of any firefighter program is to push the VT (caloric quantity) into higher intensities (caloric quality) and optimize aerobic efficiency.

When performing low-intensity training, the challenge will be focused on inspiration because there is less CO_2 produced in fat catabolism versus carbohydrate catabolism. This is why you are able to talk during a long, slow run (i.e., talk test). By improving the aerobic system, the firefighter will be able to improve their overall work capacity. High-intensity workouts will develop both inspiration and expiration of the firefighter because of the given amount of CO_2 produced and O_2 used. The body wants to remove the CO_2 by expiring forcefully and rapidly. As the intensity is increased, so does the lactate production, requiring more buffering, which produces more CO_2. When the anaerobic system improves, the firefighter will be able to continue to work at high intensity for a longer period of time.

So what is the optimal type of training for firefighters? Because most firefighters are pressed for time during their shift, a short, high-intensity, intermittent training program would be appropriate. Based on science, we know aerobic training improves the maximal aerobic power but does not change anaerobic capacity, but high-intensity intermittent training may improve both anaerobic and aerobic energy systems significantly, probably through imposing different intensities (Tabata, 1996). In another study, high-intensity training was better at increasing aerobic capacity than moderate exercise (Helgerud, 2007). However, training at low-moderate intensity is still sufficient to reduce cardiovascular risk. One study found that only one out of nineteen studies examined showed moderate-intensity exercise to be more effective than high-intensity when it came to decreasing cardiovascular health risk factors, such as high blood pressure or cholesterol, blood sugar control, or body weight (Houmard, 2004).

No conclusion has been made on the best prescription toward cardiovascular disease. Some studies found that short, intense bursts were more effective, while others found that lower intensity for longer periods of time were better (Buchan, 2011). Still, aerobic capacity is widely regarded as a good measure of physical fitness and has been shown to be a good predictor of death due to cardiovascular problems. No matter which type or intensity of exercise that the evidence deems the most effective, it will have no benefit unless the individual actually does it.

Identify the firefighter's needs first before assuming one method is the best for everyone. An older, more experienced firefighter who is overweight and has a bad back may not be inclined to do hard intervals. So apply appropriate levels of exercise and progress them along. Start them off with aerobic intervals, where specifically timed work intervals are followed by specifically timed active recovery. By applying the appropriate strategy and solution, you will help your firefighter achieve their goal, which, over time, will create a healthier department.

Physical fitness is the capacity of the heart, blood vessels, lungs, and muscles to function at optimum efficiency. There are six major components that make up physical fitness:

1.   **Cardiovascular or Aerobic Endurance**: the goal of aerobic output is to improve performance, improve health, and prevent injury. Aerobic training itself is the central feature of an effective program Aerobic output is the degree to which a firefighter can efficiently move oxygen through their body and the extent to which they can effectively utilize that oxygen will determine, in large part, how fast or long they can respond to a medical emergency or situation. By itself, increasing the training load of a firefighter doing less than thirty miles a week quite often improves aerobic performance by expanding an underdeveloped aerobic system. This increased aerobic ability creates not only additional work tolerance and better response time but also enhances the firefighter's ability to recover from highly stressful situations.

To determine aerobic capacity, many fire departments incorporate some type of aerobic assessment. The IAFF-WFI recommends the Gerkin treadmill protocol or the FDNY Stepmill test, yet many people do not have the ability to perform the test on their own.

2.   **Anaerobic Capacity:** Anaerobic training is shorter than aerobic training in duration (less than two minutes), in which oxygen is not a limiting factor in performance, and requires energy from anaerobic sources. Fire suppression is highly anaerobic and when it lasts from thirty seconds to two minutes, these physiological responses begin to rely on lactic acid (again, any activity beyond two minutes becomes aerobic training). These energy systems are effectively developed using an interval training system where the body does not fully recover between each set.

3.   **Muscular Strength**: The ability of your body's muscle to generate force in a short period of time. This type of activity relies on anaerobic energy—allowing you the short burst of energy you need to lift a heavy weight. When you increase your strength, you're often also increasing the size of your muscles as well as strengthening your connective tissues. This can help avoid injuries and, of course, make you stronger and healthier.

4.   **Muscular Endurance:** Ability to make repeated contractions against a moderate load. When your goal is muscular endurance, lift a heavy enough weight that you can only complete twelve to sixteen repetitions of each exercise.

5.   **Flexibility:** Flexibility is the ability to perform a joint action through a range of movement. Types of stretches are the following:

- Static Stretching: slow and sustained to increase movement at a particular joint when one segment is manipulated relative to another

- Passive Stretching: requires assistance from another person.

- Active Stretching: the muscle being stretched is actively moved through its ROM (range of motion). Requires greater energy than passive or static.

- Dynamic or Ballistic Stretching: refers to quick jerking and often bounce-like movements, such as bouncing when trying to touch the toes.

6.   **Mobility and Stability**: the idea of focusing on movement patterns versus muscles. As one joint is stable, another is mobile.

MOBILE	STABLE
Ankle	Knee Joint
Hip	Lumbar Region
Thoracic Spine	Sacpulo-thoracic Joint
Glenohumeral Joint	Elbow Joint

· Joint Mobility: the degree to which an articulation is allowed to move being restricted by surrounding tissues. Unrestricted movement.

· Joint Stability: the ability to maintain or control joint movement or position

· Static Stability: maintaining proper alignment without moving, while another body part is moving

· Dynamic Stability: unrestricted movement while maintaining proper alignment

· Mobility is the key, stability second. Mobility problems are movement dysfunctions.

· Loss of mobility is sometimes the only way the body can achieve some sort of stability, but it is not real. It is often looked at as stiffness or inflexibility or engineered dysfunction so you can continue to move.

7. Body Composition: The make-up of lean and fat tissue in the body. Lean tissue is composed of muscle, bone, and organs. Fat tissue is actually composed of three different categories: essential fat, storage fat, and non-essential fat. Essential and storage fat are both necessary for normal bodily function, while non-essential fat serves no real purpose.

· Good overall fitness is required for fire suppression. You should train the whole body to improve or maintain your levels of aerobic endurance, muscular strength, muscular endurance, and flexibility.

· Functional training involves performing work against resistance in such a manner that the improvements in strength directly enhance the performance of movements so that an individual's activities of daily living are easier to perform. In functional training, it is as critical to train the specific movement as it is to train the muscles involved in the movement. The brain, which controls muscular movement, thinks in terms of whole motions, not individual muscles. This will provide a more job-specific form of training in regard to fire suppression and public safety.

6

HOW TO DEVELOP AND MAINTAIN PHYSICAL FITNESS

Any physical training program has four key components that can be manipulated to produce the desired training effect. These are the mode of exercise (type of exercise, e.g., cycling, running, swimming, etc.), the training intensity (how hard you are exercising), the training duration (how long you are exercising), and the training frequency (how often you exercise). By specifically modifying these four components of training, you will be able to develop and maintain aerobic endurance, anaerobic endurance, muscular strength, muscular endurance, and flexibility. Table 1 outlines the key elements required to develop these specific components of fitness. To improve physical fitness, you will need to alter the mode, frequency, intensity, and duration of your exercise about your current level. Your training should be gradual and progressive, starting gently and building up the intensity over time. This will produce an improvement in your fitness by placing greater demands on your body.

The mode, frequency, and duration of exercise are easy to plan and monitor with a notebook and stopwatch. Setting the correct exercise intensity for muscular strength and endurance training is usually done by counting the number of repetitions that you are able to perform on a particular exercise. Most muscular strength and endurance sessions use repetition maximum (RM) as a method of setting the correct exercise intensity, the load used being specific to the particular exercise you are performing.

Intensity of aerobic exercise is more difficult to determine and hence a number of approaches to setting the correct exercise intensity are presented in Table 2. The easiest way is to rate your effort using the rating of perceived effort (RPE) scale (Borg, 1998). This scale progresses from 6 to 20, and the descriptors and example activities associated with each level will help you to relate the scale with the intensity of the activities ranging from rest (RPE 6) to maximum (RPE 20). If you have access to a heart rate monitor, the estimated heart rates associated with each RPE level are shown in the second column (not that these are typical heart rates for a typical twenty- to thirty-year-old applicant, but may vary by ten to twenty beats per minute between different individuals).

Alternatively, heart rate may also be used to set your training intensity. You will need to determine your maximum heart rate (MHR).

To calculate your MHR = 220 − age.

Due to individual variations, the predicted value is generally within ten beats of your actual maximum heart rate.

Table 1. Key elements in developing specific fitness components

	Mode	Duration	Frequency	Intensity
Cardiovascular / Aerobic Endurance	4-mile run, aerobics class, basketball, rowing, cycling	20–60 minutes	3–5 days per week	RPE 12–16 or 60–85% of MHR
Anaerobic Endurance	sprinting, circuits, intervals	20–60 minutes	1–3 days per week	RPE 17–20 or 85–100% of MHR
Muscular Strength	heavier weight training, e.g., bench press, squat	One to three sets (6–10 reps), 8–12 different exercises	2–4 days per week	60–90% repetition max (RM)
Muscular Endurance	circuit train, moderate weight training	One to three sets (10–50 reps) of 8–12 exercises	1–3 days per week	30–50% RM

Flexibility	stretching	10–30 seconds each exercise, repeated 1–3 times per muscle group or joint	2–3 days per week (daily if possible)	Move to the point of discomfort but not pain and hold, moving slightly further as the muscle relaxes.

Lippincott, Williams, and Wilkins (2000). *ACSM's Guidelines for Exercise Testing and Prescription.*

There are a number of RPE scales but the most common are the fifteen-point scale (6–20) and the nine-point scale (1–10).

Rating of Perceived Effort (RPE Scale) Level–Description	Estimated Heart Rate (beats/ min)	% Maximum Heart Rate
6–rest–lying down, sitting	<100	<50
7–very, very light–standing	<100	<50
8	<100	<50
9–very light, walking	100-120	50-60
10	100-120	50-60
11–fairly light, brisk walking	100-120	50-60
12	120-150	60-75
13–moderate, jogging	120-150	60-75
14	120-150	60-75
15–hard, steady running	150-170	75-85
16	150-170	75-85

17–very hard, fast running	170-199	85-99
18	170-199	85-99
19–very, very hard–sprinting	170-199	85-99
20–maximum effort	200	100

Source: Borg G. (1998). Borg's Perceived Exertion and Pain Scales.

7
NUTRITION

A typical firefighter's shift can be very strenuous both physically and mentally. An average shift consists of classroom time, drill ground, and physical fitness. Training is usually performed in extreme heat, carrying seventy pounds of personal protective equipment, which can cause serious fatigue and dehydration. It is important for the recruits to maintain healthy eating habits to enable them to maintain the proper energy levels throughout their training and ensure success throughout their career.

Food is made up of six nutrients: carbohydrates (sugars), fats, proteins, vitamins, minerals, and water. Basically, carbohydrates and fats are fuels for your tissues, and proteins are the building blocks and internal machinery of your cells.

FRUITS AND VEGETABLES

Fruits and vegetables are a great source of vitamins, minerals, and dietary fiber and an array of health-promoting micronutrients. A diet rich with fruits and vegetables helps reduce the risk of cancer, heart disease, high blood pressure, and diabetes. Scientific evidence says that five to nine servings of fruits and vegetables each will reduce your risk of cancer, high blood pressure, and heart disease.

Today the average US adult eats, excluding French fries, approximately 3.5 servings of fruits and vegetables per day, which means 140 million Americans are not eating the minimum daily amount of fruits and vegetables. Getting nutrients from supplements, instead of fruits and vegetables, can decrease the benefits for you over time. Supplements do not contain the variety of nutrients found in whole fruits and vegetables. In addition, high doses of single nutrients may be potentially harmful by affecting your body's ability to benefit from other health-promoting nutrients.

CARBOHYDRATES

Carbohydrates or "carbs" are made of sugar molecules. One or two sugar molecules can be linked, which are called simple sugars. Examples of simple sugars are table sugar, hard candies, and the sugars in fruits and fruit juices. When you eat simple sugars, they quickly move into your bloodstream to give you an immediate increase in blood sugar. The increase in blood sugar that occurs after eating stimulates release of insulin from your pancreas. The insulin helps move glucose into your cells.

Bread, potatoes, pasta, and rice contain complex carbohydrates, where sugar molecules are linked in long chains. Before entering your blood stream, complex carbs must be broken down in your gastrointestinal tract to simple sugars, and, as a result, their sugar molecules are released more slowly into your blood stream.

Before being used as fuel, all carbs are changed into simple sugar: glucose. Glucose is your body's "high octane" fuel. Certain of your high-performance body parts, including your brain and your muscles, during intense exercises, can only use glucose for fuel, while other cells can use fats or sugars to produce energy.

Your body stores carbohydrates in a special form of sugar known as glycogen. Glycogen stored in your liver is used to maintain your blood sugar when you are fasting. At those times, your fat cells release free fatty acids, which can be used as fuel by many of your tissues, and glucose is released from your liver to maintain your blood glucose. Your muscles require carbs to fuel intense exercise, and to provide a ready supply of energy your muscle cells also store sugars as glycogen.

FATS

Fats are a second type of fuel, and they are the major way your body stores energy. Even if you do not eat much fat, when you eat more calories than your body needs, the extra calories will be changed to fat and stored in fat cells. Fats all share the property of being organic molecules that are no soluble in water.

Dietary fats and cooking oils are compounds called triglycerides. Triglycerides are three fatty acid molecules attached to a glycerol backbone. Fatty acids occur naturally, and they differ in how long they are and in how many double bonds occur along their length.

Although fats are an efficient means to store energy, the fuel that they supply is "low octane." Your carbohydrate stores are more like a torch—the fuel that burns hot but is consumed quickly. Fats are more like candle wax. They burn a long time, but the flame is not as intense.

PROTEINS

Proteins are the building blocks of your cells, and they take part in many of the body's chemical reactions. Proteins are made of smaller molecules called amino acids. Food protein is broken down in the digestive system to these smaller molecules before being transported in your bloodstream.

There are more than twenty different amino acids. Your body makes all but nine of them, and those nine are known as essential amino acids. Animal protein (poultry, fish, meat, eggs, and milk) contain all the essential amino acids. Vegetable proteins (cereal, beans, and nuts) do not have all nine essential amino acids. Some vegetable proteins lack the essential amino acid lysine, while other lack methionine. To get all essential amino acids from vegetables, two or more complementary vegetable proteins must be combined.

The recommended amount of protein for adults is 0.8 grams for each kilograms of body weight each day or approximately one gram for each three pounds of weight.

VITAMINS AND MINERALS

Vitamins and minerals help regulate metabolism and unlock the energy stored in food. In a way, vitamins are like fuel additives that make a car's engine run smoother. There are two major kinds of vitamins: fat soluble (A, D, E, and K) and water soluble (C and the B vitamins). Most soluble vitamins cannot be stored in your body, and the extra vitamins are washed out in your urine. Fat soluble vitamins are stored in fat, and taking too much of these vitamins can build-up and cause problems. The best source of vitamins is the food you eat.

Minerals are elements that the body needs to work properly, such as iron and calcium. For example, minerals help control muscle contraction, heart rhythm, and oxygen carried in red blood cells. Minerals strengthen bones and teeth. Like with vitamins, the best source of minerals is food.

WATER AND HYDRATION

Two-thirds of your body weight is water. It is in your bloodstream and every cell. Water helps cool your body and washes out waste products. Everyone needs at least eight glasses of water each day. Physical activity causes your body to produce heat. Just like water in a car's radiator cools the engine, the fluids you drink cool your body. When you do not drink enough water fluids, your body can overheat.

In the study performed by Contreras and Espinoza (2007) of the Orange County Fire Authority, 90 percent of firefighter recruits were dehydrated before commencing a drill. It was also concluded that the body continued to rise even after several minutes of rest and recovery.

Many sports drinks are no better than water, and some fluids are worse than water. Fruit juices and soda pop have too much sugar, and the concentrated sugar solutions slow the fluid from entering your blood stream, and since they stay in your stomach longer, they can make you feel bloated.

Typical sports drinks are water plus about half the sugar in juices or soda. The lower sugar concentrations make them easier to absorb. Because water is absorbed quickly and early in exercise, sports drinks have no advantage over water. However, after about thirty minutes of intense exercise, your muscles can benefit from the sugar in sports drinks. Sports drinks also contain small amounts of salts. Although your sweat contains salt (sodium and chloride), your body has plenty of salt stores. Taking too much salt, in the form of salt tablets, can be harmful and should be avoided. Typically sports drinks can be categorized into three major types: isotonic, hypertonic, and hypotonic.

Isotonic sports drinks contain portions of water and other nutrients similar to the human body, and typically contain 6 to 8 percent carbohydrates. Most sports drinks are isotonic.

Hypertonic sports drinks contain a lesser portion of water and a greater portion of carbohydrates than the human body. A higher proportion of carbohydrates slows stomach emptying and delays hydration.

Hypotonic sports drinks contain a greater proportion of water and a lesser proportion of carbohydrates than the human body.

Energy drinks are becoming very popular within the fire department. With long hours and lack of sleep, many EMS responders are searching for other methods to stay alert. Energy drinks generally contain stimulants such as methylxanthines (including caffeine), B vitamins, and herbs. The average (eight-fluid-ounce) energy drink has about eighty milligrams of caffeine, which is roughly equivalent to one cup of coffee. Some energy drinks have as much as sixty milligrams of caffeine per ounce. Energy drinks should be consumed in moderation to avoid excessive amounts of caffeine in your system.

Energy drinks SHOULD NOT BE CONSUMED during exercise or moderate physical exertion. Caffeine acts as a diuretic, promoting dehydration and increasing the rate of removal of electrolytes.

Energy drinks often contain guarana, which is a substance chemically similar to caffeine with comparable stimulant effects. Guarana content in energy drinks must be taken into account when estimating total caffeine. Another frequent ingredient in energy drinks is ginseng, which medical experts believe interacts with and intensifies the side effects of caffeine, including nervousness, sweating, nausea, and irregular heart beat.

Most energy drinks are made of some type of carbohydrate source (glucose, maltodextrin), B vitamins, caffeine, and possibly some other minor ingredients, such as amino acids, taurine, or L-carnitine, along with some herbs. For the sake of argument, let's just focus on caffeine. A can of soda generally has about twenty-five milligrams of caffeine whereas a cup of coffee has about a hundred milligrams. A can of Red Bull will have about the same as a cup of coffee.

There are a number of studies out there with conflicting results, so let's just look at how it affects the body from a physiological point.

Every moment that you're awake, the neurons in your brain are firing away. As those neurons fire, they produce adenosine as a byproduct, but adenosine is far from excrement. Your nervous system is actively monitoring adenosine levels through receptors. Normally, when adenosine levels reach a certain point in your brain and spinal cord, your body will start nudging you toward sleep, or at least taking it easy.

Enter caffeine, and it functions as an excellent adenosine impersonator. It heads right for the adenosine receptors in your system and, because of its similarities to adenosine; it's accepted by your body as the real thing and gets into the receptors.

More importantly, caffeine actually binds to those receptors in efficient fashion, but doesn't activate them—they're plugged up by caffeine's unique shape and chemical makeup. With those receptors blocked, the brain's own stimulants, dopamine and glutamate, can do their work more freely. BUT you get wired only to the extent that your body can support. You can't use caffeine to completely wipe out an entire week's worth of very late nights of studying, but you can use it to make yourself feel less bogged down by sleepy feelings in the morning.

The effectiveness of caffeine varies significantly from person to person, due to genetics and other factors in play. The average time caffeine has before it wears off is about five to six hours. As you regularly take in caffeine, the body and mind build up a tolerance to it, so getting the same kind of boost as one's first-ever sip takes more caffeine. Over time we consume more and more, searching out that high. Eventually, the brain strives to return to its normal function while under "attack" from caffeine by up-regulating, or creating more adenosine receptors. But regular caffeine use has also been shown to decrease receptors for norepinephrine, a hormone akin to adrenaline, along with serotonin, a mood enhancer. So your caffeine may be causing the brain to change the way all of its generally excitable things are regulated. Your next Red Bull or Rockstar drink goes a little less far each time, and ends up going from an eight-ounce to a sixteen-ounce drink.

A 1995 study suggests that people become tolerant to their daily dose of caffeine—whether a single soda or a serious Rockstar habit—somewhere between a week and twelve days. Beyond the equivalent of four cups of coffee (400 mg) in your system at once, caffeine isn't giving you much more boost—in fact, at around the ten-cup level, you're probably less alert than non-drinkers. So it is recommended that you scale back on your caffeine in-take.

As stated previously, first responders work long hours, which forces them to seek out methods to stay awake: caffeine, energy drinks. But over time their bodies and brains become tolerant and therefore we drink more. Over time the body will enter a state of adrenal exhaustion. Simply put, you have pushed your adrenal glands so hard that they have burned out. By continually consuming caffeine, you are forcing your glands to secrete what they don't have, and they have to keep digging deeper and deeper, making you more and more tired over time. That's severe adrenal depletion. It doesn't take a genius to see that there might be a downside to all of this neuron activity. In fact, uncontrolled neuron-firing creates an emergency situation, which triggers the pituitary gland in the brain to secrete ACTH (adrenocorticotrophic hormone). ACTH tells the adrenal glands to pump out stress hormones—the next major side effect of caffeine.

Another side effect is the lack of sleep. For example, a firefighter may have been up all night and now it is the day time. Instead of sleeping and letting the body recover naturally, they will consume an energy drink, forcing their body to stay awake. The lack of sleep will have a significant impact on the well-being of the firefighter, such as a reduction of testosterone production and human growth hormone, increased body fat and weight, and increased risk for heart disease.

Overall, caffeine has some benefits, but if we do not control our in-take, our bodies will become tolerant. Eventually the risks will outweigh the rewards of energy drinks.

SOME THINGS YOU CAN DO TO HELP YOUR ENERGY LEVELS

- Eat a healthy breakfast with more protein in it. This will reduce the glycemic crash your get around 10:00 a.m.

- Exercise, exercise, exercise. It helps get your endorphins as well as creates more testosterone. Remember to have a snack after you are done to aid in recovery (chocolate milk is the best).

- DRINK WATER! When your body is hydrated, you will have more natural energy.

- Drink an electrolyte-containing beverage, such as a sports drink, one to two hours before you start exercising.

- When exercising, do not drink an electrolyte-containing beverage that contains more than fifty to sixty calories.

- For every pound of body weight lost during exercise, consume three eight-ounce glasses of water or electrolyte-containing beverage.

- When you lose 2 to 4 percent of your body's water, your muscular endurance will be affected.

- At 4 to 6 percent losses, you will begin to lose strength and experience heat cramps.

- At losses greater than 6 percent, you could have severe heat cramps, exhaustion, and heat stroke, which can lead to death.

APPENDIX A

Common Aerobic Equipment

Equipment	What It Does
Treadmills	Excellent for aerobic training. Builds endurance and burns many more calories than any other exercise machine, including cross-country skiers and combination upper and lower extremity exercisers
Exercycles	Very good aerobic device. Burns about 10 percent fewer calories than treadmill. Low impact with less stress on the joints, especially for those who are overweight or have arthritis.
Stair Climber	Can be excellent low-impact aerobic device when used correctly. The main problem is trying to exercise at a level too high, while supporting some of their weight on the side rails.
Elliptical Machines	Can provide excellent, low-impact conditioning for your legs. Some machines have arm levers you can use for upper extremities.
Rowers	Rowing machines offer the benefit of an all-over workout with impact on the joints. Also strengthens your upper back. Does not typically burn as many calories as a treadmill.

Cross-Country Ski Machines	Uses upper and lower extremities for total body aerobic conditioning. Does not burn as many calories as a motorized treadmill, because of lower overall exercise intensity.

APPENDIX B

PHYSICAL ASSESSMENTS

Many fire academies require a physical fitness assessment. These assessments vary from academy to academy.

1.5-MILE RUN TEST

Purpose: This test measures aerobic fitness and leg muscles endurance.

Equipment required: 1.5-mile flat and hard running course, <u>stopwatch</u>

Description/procedure: The aim of this test is to complete the 1.5-mile course in the shortest possible time. At the start, all firefighters line up behind the starting line. On the command 'go,' the clock will start, and you will begin running at your own pace. Although walking is authorized, it is   discouraged. A cool-down walk should be performed at the completion of the test

MALE (VALUES IN ML/KG/MIN)

	Poor	Below Average	Average	Above Average	Excellent	Superior
20-29	< 33.0	33 - 36.4	36.5 - **42.4**	**42.5 - 46.4**	**46.5 - 52.4**	**> 52.5**
Time (min:sec)	16:00	16:00 - 14:41	14:38 - **12:25**	**12:23 - 11:15**	**11:14 - 9:52**	**> 9:51**
METS	9.6	9.6 - 10.39	10.43 - **12.11**	**12.15 - 13.26**	13.28 -14.98	**> 15**
30-39	< 31.5	31.5 - 35.4	35.5 - 40.9	**41.0 - 44.9**	**45.0 - 49.4**	**> 49.5**
Time (min:sec)	< 17:15	17:15 - 15:08	15:09 - 12:55	**12:53 - 11:40**	**11:38 - 10:31**	**> 10:30**
METS	< 9	9 - 10.11	10.10 - 11.68	**11.71 - 12.8**	**12.86 - 14.12**	>14.14
40-49	< 30.2	30.2 - 33.5	33.6 - 38.9	**39.0 - 43.7**	**43.8 - 48.0**	**>48**

Time (min:sec)	< 18:05	18:05 - 16.06	16:02 - 13:38	**13:36 - 12:01**	**11:59 - 10:51**	**>10:51**
METS	< 8.6	8.6 - 9.57	9.60 - 11.12	**11.14 - 12.48**	**12.51 - 13.71**	**> 13.71**
50-59	< 26.1	26.1 - 30.9	31.0 - 35.7	35.8 - 40.9	**41.0 - 45.3**	**> 45.3**
Time (min:sec)	> 21:22	21.22 - 17:38	17:34 - 15:00	14:57 - 12:55	**12:53 - 11:33**	**>11:33**
METS	> 7.46	7.46 - 8.82	8.85 - 10.2	10.23 - 11.68	**11.71 - 12.94**	**> 12.94**
60+	< 20.5	20.5 - 26.0	26.1 - 32.2	32.3 -36.4	36.5 - 44.2	**> 44.2**
Time (min:sec)	> 28:25	28:25 - 21:28	21:26 - 16:50	16:48 - 14:41	14:39 - 11:52	**> 11:52**
METS	> 5.8	5.8 - 7.42	7.43 - 9.20	9.21 - 10.39	10.41 - 12.63	**> 12.63**

HIGH RISK   **LOW RISK**

FEMALE (VALUES IN ML/KG/MIN)

	Poor	Below Average	Average	Above Average	Excellent	Superior
20-29	< 23.6	23.6 -28.9	29.0 - 32.9	33.0 - 38.9	37.0 - **41.9**	**> 41.9**
Time (min:sec)	< 24:01	24:01 - 19:01	18:56 - 16:26	16:22 - 13:38	14:25 - **12:35**	**> 12:35**
METS	< 6.74	6.74 - 8.25	8.28 - 9.40	9.43 - 11.12	10.57 - **11.96**	**> 11.96**
30-39	< 22.8	22.8 - 26.9	27.0 - 31.4	31.5 - 35.6	35.7 - 40	> 40.0
Time (min:sec)	< 25:01	25:01 - 20:38	20:33 - 17:19	17:15 - 15:03	15:00 - 13:09	> 13:09
METS	< 6.5	6.5 - 7.68	7.71 - 8.96	9.0 - 10.16	10.2 - 11.49	>11.49
40-49	< 21.0	21.0 - 24.4	24.5 - 28.9	29.0 - 32.8	32.9 - 36.9	> 36.9
Time (min:sec)	< 27:36	27:36 - 23:07	23:00 - 19:01	18:56 - 16:29	16:26 - 14:33	> 14:33
METS	< 6	6 - 6.96	7 - 8.25	8.28 - 9.37	9.39 - 10.48	> 10.48
50-59	< 20.2	20.2 - 22.7	22.8 - 26.9	27.0 - 31.4	31.5 - 35.7	> 35.7
Time (min:sec)	< 28:55	28:55 - 25:09	25:01 - 20:38	20:33 - 17:10	17:15 - 15:00	> 15:00
METS	< 5.77	5.77 - 6.48	6.51 - 7.68	7.71 - 9.03	9.00 - 10.2	> 10.2
60+	< 17.5	17.5 - 20.1	20.2 - 24.4	24.5 - 30.2	30.3 - 31.4	> 31.4
Time (min:sec)	< 34:30	34:30 - 29:05	28:55 - 23:07	23:00 - 18:05	18:01 - 17:18	>17:18
METS	< 5	5.0 - 5.74	5.77 - 6.96	7.0 - 8.6	8.65 - 8.97	> 8.97

Source: The Physical Fitness Specialist Certification Manual, the Cooper Institute for Aerobics Research Dallas TX, revised 1997 printed in Advance Fitness Assessment & Exercise Prescription, 3rd Edition, Vivian H. Heyward, 1998.p48

- Firefighter should have an aerobic capacity (VO$_2$ max) of **42 ml·kg^{-1}·min^{-1}.**

- Fire recruits have a VO$_2$ max of **45 ml·kg^{-1}·min^{-1} upon entry into an academy.**

- Male Firefighters in the lowest fitness category (METS ≤ 10) had a nearly 10-fold higher prevalence of Metabolic Syndrome compared with colleagues in the highest fitness category (METS > 14) (Baur, 2011).

20-M Shuttle Test (Yo-Yo Beep Test): This test involves continuous running between two lines twenty meters apart in time to recorded beeps. For this reason, the test is also often called the 'beep' or 'bleep' test. The test subjects stand behind one of the lines facing the second line, and begin running when instructed by the CD or tape. The speed at the start is quite slow. The subject continues running between the two lines, turning when signaled by the recorded beeps. After about one minute, a sound indicates an increase in speed, and the beeps will be closer together. This continues each minute (level). If the line is not reached in time for each beep, the subject must run to the line, turn, and try to catch up with the pace within two more 'beeps.' Also, if the line is reached before the beep sounds, the subject must wait until the beep sounds. The test is stopped if the subject fails to reach the line (within two meters) for two consecutive ends.

Scoring: The athlete's score is the level and number of shuttles (twenty meters) reached before they were unable to keep up with the recording. Record the last level completed (not necessarily the level stopped at).

MALES

yrs	very poor	poor	Fair	average	good	very good	excellent
12 - 13	< 3/3	3/4 - 5/1	5/2 - 6/4	6/5 - 7/5	7/6 - 8/8	8/9 - 10/9	> 10/9
14 - 15	< 4/7	4/7 - 6/1	6/2 - 7/4	7/5 - 8/9	8/10 - 9/8	9/9 - 12/2	> 12/2
16 - 17	< 5/1	5/1 - 6/8	6/9 - 8/2	8/3 - 9/9	9/10 - 11/3	11/4 - 13/7	> 13/7
18 - 25	< 5/2	5/2 - 7/1	7/2 - 8/5	8/6 - 10/1	10/2 - 11/5	11/6 - 13/10	> 13/10
26 - 35	< 5/2	5/2 - 6/5	6/6 - 7/9	7/10 - 8/9	8/10 - 10/6	10/7 - 12/9	> 12/9
36 - 45	< 3/8	3/8 - 5/3	5/4 - 6/4	6/5 - 7/7	7/8 - 8/9	8/10 - 11/3	> 11/3
46 - 55	< 3/6	3/6 - 4/6	4/7 - 5/5	5/6 - 6/6	6/7 - 7/7	7/8 - 9/5	> 9/5
56 - 65	< 2/7	2/7 - 3/6	3/7 - 4/8	4/9 - 5/6	5/7 - 6/8	6/9 - 8/4	> 8/4
> 65	< 2/2	2/2 - 2/5	2/6 - 3/7	3/8 - 4/8	4/9 - 6/1	6/2 - 7/2	> 7/2

FEMALES

yrs	very poor	poor	Fair	average	good	very good	excellent
12 - 13	< 2/6	2/6 - 3/5	3/6 - 5/1	5/2 - 6/1	6/2 - 7/4	7/5 - 9/3	> 9/3
14 - 15	< 3/3	3/4 - 5/2	5/3 - 6/4	6/5 - 7/5	7/6 - 8/7	8/8 - 10/7	> 10/7
16 - 17	< 4/2	4/2 - 5/6	5/7 - 7/1	7/2 - 8/4	8/5 - 9/7	9/8 - 11/10	> 11/11
18 - 25	< 4/5	4/5 - 5/7	5/8 - 7/2	7/3 - 8/6	8/7 - 10/1	10/2 - 12/9	> 12/9
26 - 35	< 3/8	3/8 - 5/2	5/3 - 6/5	6/6 - 7/7	7/8 - 9/4	9/5 - 11/5	> 11/5
36 - 45	< 2/7	2/7 - 3/7	3/8 - 5/3	5/4 - 6/2	6/3 - 7/4	7/5 - 9/5	> 9/5
46 - 55	< 2/5	2/5 - 3/5	3/6 - 4/4	4/5 - 5/3	5/4 - 6/2	6/3 - 8/1	> 8/1
56 - 65	< 2/2	2/2 - 2/6	2/7 - 3/5	3/6 - 4/4	4/5 - 5/6	5/7 - 7/2	> 7/2
> 65	< 1/5	1/5 - 2/1	2/2 - 2/6	2/7 - 3/4	3/5 - 4/3	4/4 - 5/7	> 5/7

Source: (2003) The Yo-Yo Intermittent Recovery Test: Physiological Response, Reliability, and Validity. **To determine your maximum heart rate (MHR):**

Male athletes - MHR = 202 - (0.55 x age)

Female athletes - MHR = 216 - (1.09 x age)

Example: Age of 30-year-old male

202 – (0.55 x 30) = 185.5 max heart rate

MUSCULAR STRENGTH—PUSH-UPS

Purpose: Evaluation uses a series of push-ups performed in a two-minute time period (maximum of eighty push-ups).

Equipment required: Prepare five-inch prop, metronome, and stop watch.

Description/procedure: Begin in the up position (hands shoulder-width apart, back is straight, and head is in neutral position). Firefighter is not allowed to have feet against a wall or other stationary item. The back must be straight at all times, and they must push up to a straight arm position.

Perform push-ups in time with the cadence of the metronome (one beat up—one beat down).

The five-inch prop is placed on the ground beneath the client's chin, and the client must lower body to the floor until the chin touches object.

The metronome is set at a speed of eighty, allowing for forty push-ups per minute.

Termination ends when: eighty push-ups are completed, performs three consecutive incorrect push-ups, or does not maintain continuous motion with the metronome cadence.

Number of Successful Completed Push-Ups: _____

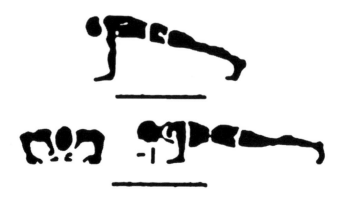

CORE MUSCULAR STRENGTH AND STABILITY TEST

Purpose: This evaluation is to monitor the development and improvements of a firefighter's core strength and endurance over time. To prepare for the assessment, you will need:

Equipment required: Prepare cushioned mat and stopwatch.

Description/procedure: Start on your hands and knees; place your forearms flat on floor with your elbows directly below your shoulders. Straighten your knees and get onto your toes so only your toes and forearms are on the floor. Hold a straight link between your neck and ankles. Be sure your back does not bow or dip.

Hold, breathing steadily—don't hold your breath!

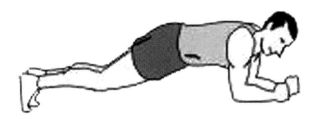

- · Under 1 minute—Needs work, keep practicing

- · 60–119 seconds—Good, keep practicing

- · 120+ seconds—Excellent

Total Time: _____

MUSCULAR STRENGTH—PULL-UPS

This is not a timed event.

Sweatshirts will be removed during the conduct of the pull-up event in order to observe the lockout of the elbows with each repetition.

Assistance to the bar with a step up, being lifted up or jumping up, is authorized. Any assistance up to the bar will not be used to continue into the first pull-up.

The bar must be grasped with both palms facing either forward or to the rear.

The correct starting position begins when the firefighter's arms are fully extended beneath the bar, feet are free from touching the ground or any bar mounting assist, and the body is motionless.

The firefighter's legs may be positioned in a straight or bent position, but may not be raised above the waist.

One repetition consists of raising the body with the arms until the chin is above the bar, and then lowering the body until the arms are fully extended; repeat the exercise. At no time during the execution of this event can a firefighter rest his chin on the bar.

The intent is to execute a vertical "dead hang" pull-up. A certain amount of inherent body movement will occur as the pull-up is executed. However, the intent is to avoid a pendulum-like motion that enhances the ability to execute the pull-up. Whipping, kicking, kipping of the body or legs, or any leg movement used to assist in the vertical progression of the pull-up is not authorized. If observed, the repetition will not count for score. To know your pull-up max, utilize the following formula:

$$\text{(Max Rep} - 1) * 0.03 = X$$

$$X * \text{Body weight} = Y$$

$$Y + \text{body weight} = \text{Max Rep}$$

*You want to be 10% of your bench press max.

A repetition will be counted when an accurate and complete pull-up is performed.

Number of Successful Completed Pull-Ups: _____

Pull body up until bar touches chin.

FLEXIBILITY—SIT AND REACH

Purpose: This is a series of three measurements that will evaluate the flexibility of the lower back, hamstring muscles, and shoulders.

Equipment required: sit-and-reach box (or alternatively a ruler can be used and held between the feet)

Description/procedure: The flexion required during evaluation must be smooth and slow, as the individual advances the slide on the box to the most distal position possible.

Sit on the floor, ensuring the head, upper back, and lower back are in contact with the wall. Keep legs together, fully extended. The sit-and-reach box is placed flat against the feet.

While maintaining head and upper/lower back contact with the wall, the client is instructed to extend arms fully in front of the body with the right hand overlaying the left hand, with middle finger of each hand directly over each other. The rule is set at 0.0 inches at the tips of the middle fingers.

Instruct the client to exhale slowly while stretching slowly forward, bending at the waist and pushing the measuring device with the middle fingers.

During the stretch, legs are to remain together and fully extended, and hands are to remain overlaid. The stretches are held momentarily and the distance obtained.

If the firefighter bounces, flexes the knees, or uses momentum to increase distance, the trial is disqualified.

Relax for thirty seconds. Records distance to the nearest one-fourth of an inch.

Conduct three trials, recording the furthest distance.

The following table is data from the American College of Sports Medicine (1995) for performance in the sit-and-reach test:

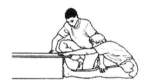

Sit and Reach Test Scores								
	Men				Women			
Percentile Rank	20-29 years		30-39 years		20-29 years		30-39 years	
	in.	cm	in.	cm	in.	cm	in.	cm
99	>23.0	>58	>22.0	>56	>24.0	>61	>24.0	>61
90	21.75	55	21.0	53	23.75	60	22.5	57
80	20.5	52	19.5	50	22.5	57	21.5	55
70	19.5	50	18.5	47	21.5	55	20.5	52
60	18.5	47	17.5	44	20.5	52	20.0	51
50	17.5	44	16.5	42	20.0	51	19.0	48
40	16.5	42	15.5	39	19.25	49	18.25	46
30	15.5	39	14.5	37	18.25	46	17.25	44
20	14.5	37	13.0	33	17.0	43	16.5	42
10	12.25	31	11.0	28	15.5	39	14.5	37
01	<10.5	<27	<9.25	<23	<14.0	<36	<12.0	<30

APPENDIX C

TYPES OF AEROBIC TRAINING

LONG, SLOW DISTANCE:

Intensity is usually less than 70 percent VO_2 max, or equivalent to about 80 percent maximum heart rate. Duration should be near to race distance or at least thirty minutes to two hours long. Intensity for long, slow distance endurance training is often gauged using the "talk" test whereby the athlete can hold a conversation without being too winded.

Adaptations to this form of aerobic endurance training include improved cardiovascular and thermoregulatory function, improved mitochondrial energy production, increased oxidative capacity of skeletal muscle, and increased utilization as fat for fuel.

PACE/TEMPO

Pace/tempo training is designed to improve energy production from both aerobic and anaerobic energy pathways. Intensity is slightly higher than race pace and corresponds to the lactate threshold. Duration is usually twenty to thirty minutes at a steady pace.

Tempo/pace training can also be performed intermittently or in intervals. Intensity is the same as steady state tempo/pace training except the session consists of a series of shorter bouts with brief recovery periods. It is important to keep intensity at or slightly higher than competition pace for either type of pace/tempo training. Progression should be in the form of increased duration rather than faster.

INTERVAL

Interval training allows the athlete to work close to their aerobic limit (VO_2 max) for a longer duration compared to a continuous type session. Short bouts of three to five minutes at an intensity close to VO_2 max are interspersed by periods of active recovery. Work to rest ratio should be 1:1 so a three-minute run should be followed by three minutes of rest.

Because this type of aerobic endurance training is very demanding, sessions should be limited both in duration and in frequency each week. Duration is usually thirty to forty-five minutes and frequency is one or two sessions per week, with ample rest days between.

REPETITION

This is the most intense form of aerobic endurance training. Performed at a pace greater than VO_2 max, it places a high demand on the anaerobic energy systems. Work intervals are usually only sixty to ninety seconds separated by rest intervals of five minutes or more. Typically work to rest ratio is 1:5.

Repetition training helps to improve running speed, running economy, and builds a greater tolerance to lactic acid. Endurance athletes often use repetition training to help in the final kick of a race. Due to the high-intensity nature, only one session per week is required.

FARTLEK

Fartlek training combines some or all of the above aerobic endurance training techniques. A long, slow run/cycle (at about 70 percent VO_2 max) forms the foundation of the session and is combined with short bursts of higher intensity work. There is no set format for a Fartlek session although there are some standard sessions that have been developed by coaches over the years. Fartlek endurance training will improve VO_2 max, exercise economy, and lactate threshold. It also adds a nice change of pace to the more monotonous steady-state training.

THE TEN-PERCENT RULE

Increasing the intensity, time, or type of activity too quickly is one common reason for sport injury. To prevent this, many fitness experts recommend that both novice and expert athletes follow the ten-percent rule, which sets a limit on increases in weekly training. This guideline simply states that you should increase your activity no more than 10 percent per week. That includes distance, intensity, weight lifted, and time of exercise.

APPENDIX D

CANDIDATE PHYSICAL AGILITY TEST (CPAT) PREPARATION GUIDE

The Fire Service Joint Labor Management Wellness/Fitness Initiative Candidate Physical Ability Test© consists of eight separate events. The CPAT is a sequence of events requiring the candidate to progress along a predetermined path from event to event in a continuous manner. This test was developed to allow fire departments a means for obtaining pools of trainable candidates who are physically able to perform essential job tasks at fire scenes.

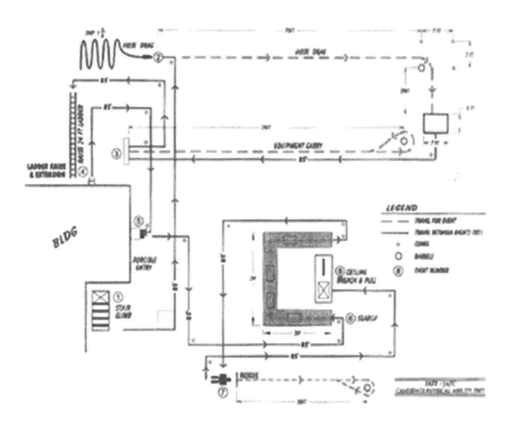

The CPAT consist of the following eight events:

- Stair Climb: For this event, you must wear two 12.5-pound weights on your shoulders to simulate the weight of a high-rise pack. Prior to the initiations of the timed CPAT, there is a twenty-second warm-up on the StepMill at a set stepping rate of fifty steps per minute. During this warm-up period, you are permitted to dismount, grasp the rail, or hold the wall to establish balance and cadence. If you fall or dismount the StepMill during the twenty-second warm-up period, you must remount the StepMill and restart the entire twenty-second warm-up period. You are allowed to restart the warm-up period twice. The timing of the test begins at the end of this warm-up period when the proctor calls, "Start." There is no break in time between the warm-up period and the actual timing of the test. For the test, you must walk on the StepMill at a set stepping rate of sixty steps per minute for three minutes. This concludes the event. The two 12.5-pound weights are removed from your shoulders. Walk eighty-five feet within the established walkway to the next event.

- Hose Drag: For this event, you must grasp a hoseline nozzle attached to two hundred feet of 1¾-inch hose. Place the hoseline over your shoulder or across your chest, not exceeding the eight-foot mark. You are permitted to run during the hose drag. Drag the hose seventy-five feet to a pre-positioned drum, make a ninety-degree turn around the drum, and continue an additional twenty-five feet. Stop within the marked five-foot-by-seven-foot box, drop to at least one knee, and pull the hoseline until the hoseline fifty-foot mark crosses the finish line. During the hose pull, you must keep at least one knee in contact with the ground and knee(s) must remain within the marked boundary lines. This concludes the event. Walk eighty-five feet within the established walkway to the next event.

- Equipment Carry: For this event, you must remove the two saws from the tool cabinet, one at a time, and place them on the ground and adjust your grip. Upon return to the tool cabinet, place the saws on the ground, pick up each saw one at a time, and replace the saw in the designated space in the cabinet. This concludes the event. Walk eighty-five feet within the established walkway to the next event.

- Ladder Raise and Extension: For this event, you must walk to the top rung of the twenty-four-foot aluminum extension ladder, lift the unhinged end from the ground, and walk it up until it is stationary against the wall. This must be done in a hand-over-hand fashion, using each rung until the ladder is stationary against the wall. You must not use the ladder rails to raise the ladder. Immediately proceed to the pre-positioned and secured twenty-four-foot aluminum extension ladder, stand with both feet within the marked box of thirty-six inches by thirty-six inches, and extend the fly section hand over hand until it hits the stop. Then, lower the fly section hand over hand in a controlled fashion to the starting position. This concludes the event. Walk eighty-five feet within the established walkway to the next event.

· Forcible Entry: For this event, you must use a ten-pound sledgehammer to strike the measuring device in the target area until the buzzer is activated. During this event, you must keep your feet outside the toe-box at all times. After the buzzer is activated, place the sledgehammer on the ground. This concludes the event. Walk eighty-five feet within the established walkway to the next event.

· Search: For this event, you must crawl through a tunnel maze that is approximately three feet high, four feet wide, and sixty-four feet in length with two ninety-degree turns. At a number of locations in the tunnel, you must navigate around, over, and under obstacles. In addition, at two locations, you must crawl through a narrowed space where the dimensions of the tunnel are reduced. Your movement is monitored through the maze. If for any reason you choose to end the event, call or rap sharply on the wall or ceiling and you will be assisted out of the maze. Upon exit from the maze, the event is concluded. Walk eighty-five feet within the established walkway to the next event.

· Rescue Drag: For this event, you must grasp a 165-pound mannequin by the handle(s) on the shoulder(s) of the harness (either one or both handles are permitted), drag it thirty-five feet to a pre-positioned drum, make a 180-degree turn around the drum, and continue an additional thirty-five feet to the finish line. You are not permitted to grasp or rest on the drum. It is permissible for the mannequin to touch the drum. You are permitted to drop and release the mannequin and adjust your grip. The entire mannequin must be dragged until it crosses the marked finish line. This concludes the event. Walk eighty-five feet within the established walkway to the next event.

- Ceiling Pull: For this event, you must remove the pike pole from the bracket, stand within the boundary established by the equipment frame, and place the tip of the pole on the painted area of the hinged door in the ceiling. Fully push up the sixty-pound hinged door in the ceiling with the pike pole three times. Then, hook the pike pole to the eighty-pound ceiling device and pull the pole down five times. Each set consists of three pushes and five pulls. Repeat the set four times. You are permitted to stop and, if needed, adjust your grip. Releasing your grip or allowing the pike pole handle to slip, without the pike pole falling to the ground, does not result in a warning or constitute a failure. You are permitted to re-establish your grip and resume the event. If you do not successfully complete a repetition, the proctor calls out, "Miss" and you must push or pull the apparatus again to complete the repetition. This event and the total test time ends when you complete the final pull stroke repetition or as indicated by a proctor who calls out, "Time."

APPENDIX E

TRAINING WITH A FORTY-EIGHT/NINETY-SIX SHIFT SCHEDULE

REST AND RECOVERY: THE FORGOTTEN TRAINING CONCEPT

Training is a key component for any athlete. As a firefighter, you understand how improved power, strength, or whatever parameter you are working on will benefit you in becoming operationally fit. You understand that training will help you improve in these areas to allow you to maintain a high level of operational readiness. The question is: when do all the sets and repetitions pay off? When do the adaptations occur? Is more better? These adaptations occur during recovery, which is why recovery is such a vital component to your training. However, recovery often is not seen as important. In reality, the bottom line is that without proper recovery, your body will not achieve all the potential benefits from training.

So how do you determine how to get the proper recovery, yet still maintain a healthy lifestyle? The amount of recovery time required between workouts depends on several variables. These variables include: training history, training intensity, volume, and program goals.

As more years of training are accumulated, less recovery time is needed because the body has adapted to the training. However, as a firefighter gets older (forties to fifties), the more time is needed to recover. Beginners require more recovery time than experienced athletes. Beginners should train with forty-eight hours of recovery between strength training sessions. A program with this type of frequency lends itself nicely to a forty-eight/ninety-six work schedule.

Example: Sample of Forty-eight/Ninety-six Schedule

Monday (1st, 24-hour shift)	Tuesday (2nd, 24-hour shift)	Wednesday OFF	Thursday OFF	Friday OFF	Saturday OFF	Sunday (1st, 24-hour shift)
Light Weights	Light Cardio	Medium Weights	Light Cardio	Heavy Weights		Light Weights
2 Sets		3 Sets		4 Sets		2 Sets
12–15 Reps		8–10 Reps		6–8 Reps		12–15 Reps
Olympic (DB Clean)		Olympic (Clean)		Olympic (Clean)		Olympic (DB Clean)
Squat (Leg)		Squat (Leg)		Squat (Leg)		Squat (Leg)
Pull (Pull- Up)		Pull		Pull		Pull (Pull- Up)
Press (DB Bench)		Press (Incline Bench)		Press (Flat Bench)		Press (DB Bench)
Pull (Row)		Pull (DB Row)		Pull		Pull (Row)
Push (Alt DB Curl to Press)		Push (Military Press)		Push		Push (Alt DB Curl to Press)

More experienced athletes require higher intensities and volumes to continue seeing gains with training. As training experience, intensity, and volume increase, so should recovery time. As a result, experienced athletes may train with seventy-two hours of recovery between workouts of the same muscle group.

This is the key to building more time into workout sessions. Beginners only require forty-eight hours of recovery between workout, and they are most likely performing full-body workouts. The advanced athlete requires more frequency, intensity, and volume to achieve their goals, while working with a larger recovery period. So their workouts are divided or split so that opposing muscles groups or body parts are targeted on consecutive days.

For example, a common split is to perform upper-body exercises on Monday and Thursday and lower-body exercises on Tuesday and Friday. This provides four training days per week. Although each area is only targeted twice per week with the beginners program, more time is available to train each area. Now there is more time in each training session since only half of the body is targeted that day. This way more exercise, or higher volume and intensities, can be used. Additionally, longer rest periods can be used in between sets.

Monday (1st, 24-hour shift)	Tuesday (2nd, 24-hour shift)	Wednesday OFF	Thursday OFF	Friday OFF	Saturday OFF	Sunday (1st, 24-hour shift)
Light Cardio	Light Weights	Heavy Weights		Heavy Weights	Medium Weights	Light Cardio
	2 Sets	4 Sets		4 Sets	3 Sets	
	12–15 Reps	6–8 Reps		6–8 Reps	8–10 Reps	
	Pull-Up	Olympic (Cleans)		Pull-Up	Olympic (DB Cleans)	
	DB Bench/ Incline Press	Squat (Legs)		Flat Bench	Squat (Legs)	
	Row (Back)	Hamstrings (RDL)		Row (Back)	Hamstrings (RDL)	
	Press	Leg Ext		Press	Leg Ext	

This four-day split provides seventy-two hours of recovery between upper-body exercises. Additionally, it will provide seventy-two hours of recovery between lower-body exercises. This longer recovery time is vital for adaptations to occur with advanced programs.

Program goals also affect recovery. With a program that places you in a phase of training where the goal is to improve power (such as pre-season), then the training intensity should be very high as well. With a program that places you in a phase of training, the goal is maintenance, not improvement, and intensity and volume should decrease. Consequently, less recovery is needed when the goal is maintenance. Although it does little good to recover so rapidly from a workout that may not be repeated for a week, it does play a part when complete recovery from a workout is needed for executing operations.

APPENDIX F

DYNAMIC WARM-UP

Created By: John Hofman

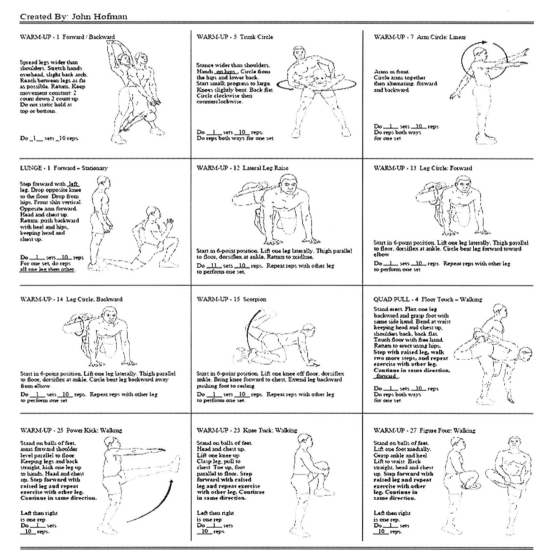

WARM-UP - 1 Forward / Backward

Spread legs wider than shoulders. Stretch hands overhead, slight back arch. Reach between legs as far as possible. Return. Keep movement constant: 2 count down 2 count up. Do not static hold at top or bottom.

Do _1_ sets _10_ reps.

WARM-UP - 5 Trunk Circle

Stance wider than shoulders. Hands on hips. Circle from the hips and lower back. Start small; progress to large. Knees slightly bent. Back flat. Circle clockwise then counterclockwise.

Do _1_ sets _10_ reps. Do reps both ways for one set

WARM-UP - 7 Arm Circle: Linear

Arms in front. Circle arms together then alternating: forward and backward

Do _1_ sets _10_ reps. Do reps both ways for one set.

LUNGE - 1 Forward - Stationary

Step forward with _left_ leg. Drop opposite knee to the floor. Drop from hips. Front shin vertical. Opposite arm forward. Head and chest up. Return: push backward with heel and hips, keeping head and chest up.

Do _1_ sets _10_ reps. For one set, do reps all one leg then other.

WARM-UP - 12 Lateral Leg Raise

Start in 6-point position. Lift one leg laterally. Thigh parallel to floor, dorsiflex at ankle. Return to midline.

Do _11_ sets _10_ reps. Repeat reps with other leg to perform one set.

WARM-UP - 13 Leg Circle: Forward

Start in 6-point position. Lift one leg laterally. Thigh parallel to floor, dorsiflex at ankle. Circle bent leg forward toward elbow

Do _1_ sets _10_ reps. Repeat reps with other leg to perform one set

WARM-UP - 14 Leg Circle: Backward

Start in 6-point position. Lift one leg laterally. Thigh parallel to floor, dorsiflex at ankle. Circle bent leg backward away from elbow

Do _1_ sets _10_ reps. Repeat reps with other leg to perform one set

WARM-UP - 15 Scorpion

Start in 6-point position. Lift one leg off floor, dorsiflex ankle. Bring knee forward to chest. Extend leg backward pushing foot to ceiling.

Do _1_ sets _10_ reps. Repeat reps with other leg to perform one set.

QUAD PULL - 4 Floor Touch - Walking

Stand erect. Flex one leg backward and grasp foot with same side hand. Bend at waist keeping head and chest up, shoulders back, back flat. Touch floor with free hand. Return to erect using hips. Step with raised leg, walk two more steps, and repeat exercise with other leg. Continue in same direction. _forward_

Do _1_ sets _10_ reps Do reps both ways for one set

WARM-UP - 25 Power Kick: Walking

Stand on balls of feet. arms forward shoulder level parallel to floor. Keeping legs and back straight, kick one leg up to hands. Head and chest up. Step forward with raised leg and repeat exercise with other leg. Continue in same direction.

Left then right is one rep Do _1_ sets _10_ reps.

WARM-UP - 23 Knee Tuck: Walking

Stand on balls of feet. Head and chest up. Lift one knee up Clasp leg, pull to chest Toe up, foot parallel to floor. Step forward with raised leg and repeat exercise with other leg. Continue in same direction.

Left then right is one rep Do _1_ sets _10_ reps.

WARM-UP - 27 Figure Four: Walking

Stand on balls of feet. Lift one foot medially. Grasp ankle and heel Lift to waist. Back straight, head and chest up. Step forward with raised leg and repeat exercise with other leg. Continue in same direction.

Left then right is one rep Do _1_ sets _10_ reps.

Page 1 of 1

APPENDIX G

DETERMINE YOUR TARGET HEART RATE (THR):

Zone 1 **(50–60% of MHR)**	The lowest level you can exercise in and still increase fitness levels. For beginners or people who have not exercised for a long period of time. This zone can be for just improving your overall health. It can also be a good recovery zone for people who are over-training and need to take a break.
Zone 2 **(60–70% of MHR)**	This is the zone where the heart begins to benefit. Training in this zone will begin to improve your hearts ability to pump blood and improve the muscle cells' ability to utilize oxygen.
Zone 3 **(70–80% of MHR)**	This zone is the most effective for overall cardiovascular fitness and is often called the "aerobic zone" or "target heart rate zone." This is the optimal zone to workout in to increase your cardio-respiratory capacity or the body's ability to transport oxygenated blood to the muscle cells and carbon dioxide away from the cells.
Zone 4 **(80–90% of** **MHR) (85–90%** **= Anaerobic** **Threshold)**	This level is where you cross over from aerobic training to anaerobic training, which is called the anaerobic threshold or AT. This is the point where the body cannot effectively remove lactic acid from the working muscles quickly enough. Lactic acid is a byproduct of glycogen consumption by the working muscles. This zone is primarily for people who want to increase their performance levels.
Zone 5 **(90–100% of MHR)** **(VO$_2$ Max)**	You will only be able to train in this zone for short periods of time. You should not train at this level unless you are very fit. In this zone lactic acid develops very quickly as you are operating with oxygen debt to the muscles.

APPENDIX H

SMART GOAL SETTING—A SUREFIRE WAY TO ACHIEVE YOUR GOALS

S = Specific goal has a much greater chance of being accomplished than a general goal. To set a specific goal, you must answer the six "W" questions:

*Who: Who is involved?

*What: What do I want to accomplish?

*Where: Identify a location.

*When: Establish a timeframe.

*Which: Identify requirements and constraints.

*Why: Specific reasons, purpose, or benefits of accomplishing the goal

M = Measurable Establish concrete criteria for measuring progress toward the attainment of each goal you set. When you measure your progress, you stay on track, reach your target dates, and experience the exhilaration of achievement that spurs you on to continued effort required to reach your goal.

A = Attainable When you identify goals that are most important to you, you begin to figure out ways you can make them come true. You develop the attitudes, abilities, skills, and financial capacity to reach them. You begin seeing previously overlooked opportunities to bring yourself closer to the achievement of your goals.

R = Realistic To be realistic, a goal must represent an objective toward which you are both *willing* and *able* to work.

T = Timely A goal should be grounded within a timeframe. With no timeframe tied to it, there's no sense of urgency.

Setting goals is more than deciding what you want to do. It involves figuring out what you need to do to get where you want to go and how long it will take you to get there. Now you know the fundamentals of goal-setting. Keep the SMART acronym in mind to help you remember the basics. The next step is translating this process to fit your needs.

HOW IT WORKS

First, perform the selected fitness assessments in the following order *(see Appendix____):*

RESULTS

1. 1.5-Mile Run   _____

2. Pull-Ups   _____

3. Core Strength and Stability: Plank   _____

4. Push-Up with Metronome (80 bpm)   _____

Now score your results based on each category:

	5 points Optimal	4 points Recommended	3 points Marginal	2 points Inadequate
Aerobic Capacity 1.5-Mile Run	Under 10:20	10:21–11:29	11:30–13:14	13:15 or higher
Muscular Strength Pull-Ups	15 or higher	11–15	5–10	4 or less
Plank	120 + seconds	119–90 seconds	89–60 seconds	< 59 seconds
Push-Ups (80 bpm)	56 or higher	45 – 55	35–45	34 or less

	RESULTS	POINTS
1. 1.5-Mile Run	_____	_____
2. Pull-Ups	_____	_____
3. Plank	_____	_____
4. Push-Up with Metronome (80 bpm)	_____	_____

TOTAL SCORE _____

Once you have your total score, you can start at the proper level of training.

8–11 total points	BEGINNER LEVEL
12–15 total points	INTERMEDIATE LEVEL
16–20 total points	ADVANCED LEVEL

Example:	TOTALS	POINTS
1.5-mile run was completed in	11:27	4
Pull-Ups:	3	2
Curl-Ups:	25	2
Push-Ups:	44	4
TOTAL POINTS		**12**

This individual would start with the **intermediate level program.**

Once you have completed your selected program, re-assess yourself; if you have improved, move on to the next level of training.

Make sure to adhere to safe training protocols outlined in the manual, always check with your health provider first before starting any type of exercise program, and **NEVER PUSH YOURSELF INTO HARM'S WAY...TRAIN SMARTER, NOT HARDER!**

Weight Training Program	
BEGINNER PROGRAM	
Week: 1	

DAY ONE	**Instructions:** Short Interval Training	
Exercise		

Warm Up: 3 minute Jump Rope + Dynamic Warm Up (see Appendix F)

Cardio: Select any of the following: Running (ie treadmill), Air Dyne Bike, Rowing Machine and Perform the following workout.

Sprint for 20 seconds at Zone 3 (hard), then walk/rest for 40 seconds at Zone 1 (easy) for a total of 20 minutes.
Work to Rest Ratio: 1:2 Intensity: Hard-Easy - once you have completed the cardio portion, move onto the following:
Leg Complex I: Body Weight Squats for 20 Seconds, followed by Squat Jumps for 20 seconds, followed by Squat Holds for 20 seconds. rest 2 minutes. Perform 3 rounds. **Pull Ups:** 1-1-2-2-2-1-1 rest 30 seconds between each set: total reps 10 **Push Ups:** 8-8-9-9-10-9-9-8-8 reps / rest 45 seconds in between each set: 78 total reps
Cool Down: Walk Easy for 5 minutes and perform static stretching

DAY TWO & FIVE	**Instructions: Giant Set: A combination of exercises performed in order with little or no rest in between. For example: Squat, Pull Up, Push Up, Plank......once you have completed a round you start over again.**	

	Exercise:	**Set 1**		**Set 2**		**Set 3**		**Set 4**		**Set 5**		**Set 6**		**Total lbs**
		Reps	**lbs**	**Reps**	**lbs**	**Reps**	**lbs**	**Reps**	**lbs**	**Reps**	**lbs**	**Reps**	**lbs**	**lifted /**
1	Split Squat	15		15										
2	Inverted Pull Up	15		15										
3	Dumbbell (DB) Bench Press	15		15										
4	Plank Row: each side (es)	15		15										
5	DB Alt Curl to Press (es)	15		15										
6	Double Leg (DL) Pelvic Lift	15		15										
7	Plank (hold for time)	10 sec		10 sec										
8	Modfied Side Plank (es)	10 sec		10 sec										
9	Mt Climber (es)	15		15										
	Totals	105	0	105	0	0	0	0	0	0	0	0	0	0

DAY THREE, SIX AND SEVEN:	**REST DAY (Stratic Strech, Self Myo-Fascial Release Techniques)**

DAY FOUR	**Instructions:** Long Interval Training	
Exercise		

Warm Up: 3 minute Jump Rope + Dynamic Warm Up (see Appendix F)

Cardio: Select any of the following: Running (ie treadmill), Air Dyne Bike, Rowing Machine and Perform the following workout.

Exercise for moderate pace for 1 minute at Zone 2- 3 (medium/hard), then walk/rest for 1 minute at Zone 1 (easy) for a total of 20 minutes.Work to Rest Ratio: 1:1 Intensity: Hard-Easy - once you have completed the cardio portion, move onto the following:
Leg Complex II: 20 Body Weight Squats, immediatley 20 split jumps, 10 body weight squats. rest 2 minutes between each round. Perform 3 rounds **Pull Ups:** 1-1-2-2-2-1-1 rest 30 seconds between each set: total reps 10 **Push Ups:** 8-8-9-9-10-9-9-8-8 reps / rest

Cool Down: Walk Easy for 5 minutes and perform static stretching

Weight Training Program			
ADVANCED PROGRAM			
Week: 2			

DAY ONE	Instructions: Short Interval Training
Exercise	

Warm Up: 3 minute Jump Rope + Dynamic Warm Up (see Appendix F)

Cardio: Select any of the following: Running (ie treadmill), Air Dyne Bike, Rowing Machine and Perform the following workout.

Sprint for 20 seconds at Zone 3 (hard), then walk/rest for 10 seconds at Zone 1 (easy) for a total of 24 minutes. Work to Rest Ratio: 1:1 Intensity: Hard-Easy - once you have completed the cardio portion, move onto the following: **Leg Complex I:** Body Weight Squats for 20 Seconds, followed by Squat Jumps for 20 seconds, followed by Squat Holds for 20 seconds. rest 30 seconds. Perform 4 rounds. **Pull Ups:** 8-8-9-9-10-9-9-8-8 rest 30 seconds between each set: total reps 78 **Push Ups:** 13-13-14-14-15-14-14-13-13 reps / rest 45 seconds in between each set: 123 total reps

Cool Down: Walk Easy for 5 minutes and perform static stretching

DAY TWO & FIVE	Instructions: Super Giant Set: A combination of exercises performed in order with little or no rest in between. For example: Squat, Pull Up, Push Up, Plank.......once you have completed a round you start over again.

	Exercise:	Set 1		Set 2		Set 3		Set 4		Set 5		Set 6		Total lbs
		Reps	lbs	Reps	lbs	Reps	lbs	Reps	lbs	Reps	lbs	Reps	lbs	lifted / ex.
1a	Elevated Foot Squat	12		12		12								
1b	Squat Jump	5		5		5								
2a	Inverted Pull Up	12		12		12								
2b	Plank Row: each side (es)	5		5		5								
3a	Dumbbell (DB) Bench Press	12		12		12								
3b	Clap Push Up	5		5		5								
4	Physioball Punch	12		12		12								
5a	DB Alt Curl to Press (es)	12		12		12								
5b	Spider Push Up (es)	12		12		12								
6	Physioball Glute Ham	12		12		12								
7	Stir the Pot (each direction)	12		12		12								
8	Palloof Press (es)	10 sec		10 sec		10 sec								
9	Mt Climber with Push Up (es)	10 sec		10 sec		10 sec								
	Totals	99	0	99	0	99	0	0		0		0		0

DAY THREE, SIX AND SEVEN:	REST DAY (Stratic Strech, Self Myo-Fascial Release Techniques)

DAY FOUR	Instructions: Long Interval Training
Exercise	

Warm Up: 3 minute Jump Rope + Dynamic Warm Up (see Appendix F)

Cardio: Select any of the following: Running (ie treadmill), Air Dyne Bike, Rowing Machine and Perform the following workout.

Exercise for moderate pace for 1:30 minute at Zone 2- 3 (medium/hard), then walk/rest for 30 seconds at Zone 1 (easy) for a total of 24 minutes. Work to Rest Ratio: 1.5:1 Intensity: Hard-Easy - once you have completed the cardio portion, move onto the following: **Leg Complex II:** 20 Body Weight Squats, immediatley 20 split jumps, 10 body weight squats. rest 15 seconds between each round. Perform 4 rounds **Pull Ups:** 8-8-9-9-10-9-9-8-8 rest 30 seconds between each set: total reps 78 **Push Ups:** 13-13-14-14-15-14-14-13-13 reps / rest 45 seconds in between each set: 123 total reps

Cool Down: Walk Easy for 5 minutes and perform static stretching

Weight Training Program	
BEGINNER PROGRAM	
Week: 3	

DAY ONE	Instructions: Short Interval Training
Exercise	

Warm Up: 3 minute Jump Rope + Dynamic Warm Up (see Appendix F)

Cardio: Select any of the following: Running (ie treadmill), Air Dyne Bike, Rowing Machine and Perform the following workout.

Sprint for 20 seconds at Zone 3 (hard), then walk/rest for 40 seconds at Zone 1 (easy) for a total of 30 minutes.
Work to Rest Ratio: 1:2 Intensity: Hard-Easy - once you have completed the cardio portion, move onto the following:
Leg Complex I: Body Weight Squats for 20 Seconds, followed by Squat Jumps for 20 seconds, followed by Squat Holds for 20 seconds. rest 2 minutes. Perform 5 rounds. **Pull Ups:** 1-2-2-3-3-2-2-1 rest 30 seconds between each set: total reps 16
Push Ups: 8-9-10-10-11-11-10-10-9-8 reps / rest 45 seconds in between each set: 96 total reps

Cool Down: Walk Easy for 5 minutes and perform static stretching

DAY TWO & FIVE	Instructions: Giant Set: A combination of exercises performed in order with little or no rest in between. For example: Squat, Pull Up, Push Up, Plank......once you have completed a round you start over again.												
Exercise:	Set 1		Set 2		Set 3		Set 4		Set 5		Set 6		Total lbs lifted /
	Reps	lbs	Reps	lbs	Reps	lbs	Reps	lbs	Reps	lbs	Reps	lbs	
1 Split Squat	10		10		10		10						
2 Inverted Pull Up	10		10		10		10						
3 Dumbbell (DB) Bench Press	10		10		10		10						
4 Plank Row: each side (es)	10		10		10		10						
5 DB Alt Curl to Press (es)	10		10		10		10						
6 Double Leg (DL) Pelvic Lift	10		10		10		10						
7 Plank (hold for time)	10 sec		10 sec		10 sec		10 sec						
8 Modfied Side Plank (es)	10 sec		10 sec		10 sec		10 sec						
9 Mt Climber (es)	10		10		10		10						
Totals	70	0	70	0	70	0	70	0	0	0	0	0	0

DAY THREE, SIX AND SEVEN:	REST DAY (Stratic Strech, Self Myo-Fascial Release Techniques)

DAY FOUR	Instructions: Long Interval Training
Exercise	

Warm Up: 3 minute Jump Rope + Dynamic Warm Up (see Appendix F)

Cardio: Select any of the following: Running (ie treadmill), Air Dyne Bike, Rowing Machine and Perform the following workout.

Exercise for moderate pace for 1 minute at Zone 2- 3 (medium/hard), then walk/rest for 1 minute at Zone 1 (easy) for a total of 28 minutes. Work to Rest Ratio: 1:1 Intensity: Hard-Easy - once you have completed the cardio portion, move onto the following:
Leg Complex II: 20 Body Weight Squats, immediatley 20 split jumps, 10 body weight squats. rest 2 minutes between each round. Perform 5 rounds **Pull Ups:** 1-2-2-3-3-2-2-1 rest 30 seconds between each set: total reps 16 **Push Ups:** 8-9-10-10-11-11-10-10-9-8 reps / rest 45 seconds in between each set: 96 total reps

Cool Down: Walk Easy for 5 minutes and perform static stretching

Weight Training Program		
BEGINNER PROGRAM		
Week: 4		

DAY ONE	Instructions: Short Interval Training	
Exercise		

Warm Up: 3 minute Jump Rope + Dynamic Warm Up (see Appendix F)

Cardio: Select any of the following: Running (ie treadmill), Air Dyne Bike, Rowing Machine and Perform the following workout.

Sprint for 30 seconds at Zone 3 (hard), then walk/rest for 30 seconds at Zone 1 (easy) for a total of 20 minutes.
Work to Rest Ratio: 1:1 Intensity: Hard-Easy - once you have completed the cardio portion, move onto the following:
Leg Complex I: Body Weight Squats for 20 Seconds, followed by Squat Jumps for 20 seconds, followed by Squat Holds for 20 seconds. rest 1 minutes. Perform 3 rounds. **Pull Ups:** 2-2-3-3-4-3-3-2-2 rest 30 seconds between each set: total reps 24
Push Ups: 9-9-10-10-11-11-12-11-11-10-10-9-9 reps / rest 45 seconds in between each set: 110 total reps

Cool Down: Walk Easy for 5 minutes and perform static stretching

DAY TWO & FIVE	Instructions: Giant Set: A combination of exercises performed in order with little or no rest in between. For example: Squat, Pull Up, Push Up, Plank......once you have												
Exercise:	**Set 1**		**Set 2**		**Set 3**		**Set 4**		**Set 5**		**Set 6**		**Total lbs**
	Reps	lbs	Reps	lbs	Reps	lbs	Reps	lbs	Reps	lbs	Reps	lbs	lifted /
1 Split Squat	8		8		8		8						
2 Inverted Pull Up	8		8		8		8						
3 Dumbbell (DB) Bench Press	8		8		8		8						
4 Plank Row: each side (es)	8		8		8		8						
5 DB Alt Curl to Press (es)	8		8		8		8						
6 Double Leg (DL) Pelvic Lift	8		8		8		8						
7 Plank (hold for time)	10 sec		10 sec		10 sec		10 sec						
8 Side Plank (es)	10 sec		10 sec		10 sec		10 sec						
9 Mt Climber (es)	8		8		8		8						
Totals	56	0	56	0	56	0	56	0	0	0	0	0	0

DAY THREE, SIX AND SEVEN:	REST DAY (Stratic Strech, Self Myo-Fascial Release Techniques)

DAY FOUR	Instructions: Long Interval Training
Exercise	

Warm Up: 3 minute Jump Rope + Dynamic Warm Up (see Appendix F)
Cardio: Select any of the following: Running (ie treadmill), Air Dyne Bike, Rowing Machine and Perform the following workout.

Exercise for moderate pace for 2 minute at Zone 2- 3 (medium/hard), then walk/rest for 1 minute at Zone 1 (easy) for a total of 21

Cool Down: Walk Easy for 5 minutes and perform static stretching

Weight Training Program	
BEGINNER PROGRAM	
Week: 5	
RECOVERY	

DAY ONE	Instructions: Short Interval Training
Exercise	

Warm Up: 3 minute Jump Rope + Dynamic Warm Up (see Appendix F)

Cardio: Select any of the following: Running (ie treadmill), Air Dyne Bike, Rowing Machine and Perform the following workout.

Sprint for 30 seconds at Zone 3 (hard), then walk/rest for 30 seconds at Zone 1 (easy) for a total of 15 minutes.

Cool Down: Walk Easy for 5 minutes and perform static stretching

DAY TWO & FIVE	Instructions: Giant Set: A combination of exercises performed in order with little or no rest in between. For example: Squat, Pull Up, Push Up, Plank......once you have completed a round you start over again.

Exercise:	Set 1 Reps	lbs	Set 2 Reps	lbs	Set 3 Reps	lbs	Set 4 Reps	lbs	Set 5 Reps	lbs	Set 6 Reps	lbs	Total lbs lifted /
1 Split Squat	10		10										
2 Inverted Pull Up	10		10										
3 Dumbbell (DB) Bench Press	10		10										
4 Plank Row: each side (es)	10		10										
5 DB Alt Curl to Press (es)	10		10										
6 Double Leg (DL) Pelvic Lift	10		10										
7 Plank (hold for time)	10 sec		10 sec										
8 Side Plank (es)	10 sec		10 sec										
9 Mt Climber (es)	10		10										
Totals	70	0	70	0	0	0	0	0	0	0	0	0	

DAY THREE, SIX AND SEVEN:	REST DAY (Stratic Strech, Self Myo-Fascial Release Techniques)

DAY FOUR	Instructions: Long Interval Training
Exercise	

Warm Up: 3 minute Jump Rope + Dynamic Warm Up (see Appendix F)

Cardio: Select any of the following: Running (ie treadmill), Air Dyne Bike, Rowing Machine and Perform the following workout.

Exercise for moderate pace for 1 minute at Zone 2- 3 (medium/hard), then walk/rest for 1 minute at Zone 1 (easy) for a total of 14 minutes. Work to Rest Ratio: 2:1 Intensity: Hard-Easy - once you have completed the cardio portion, move onto the following:
Leg Complex II: 20 Body Weight Squats, immediatley 20 split jumps, 10 body weight squats. rest 1 minutes between each round. Perform 3 rounds **Pull Ups:** 2-2-3-3-4-3-3-2-2 rest 30 seconds between each set: total reps 24 **Push Ups:** 9-9-10-10-11-11-12-11-11-10-10-9-9 reps / rest 45 seconds in between each set: 110 total reps

Cool Down: Walk Easy for 5 minutes and perform static stretching

YOU HAVE COMPLETED THE BEGINNERS LEVEL. GIVE YOURSELF A THE WEEKEND OFF AND RE-TEST YOURSELF.

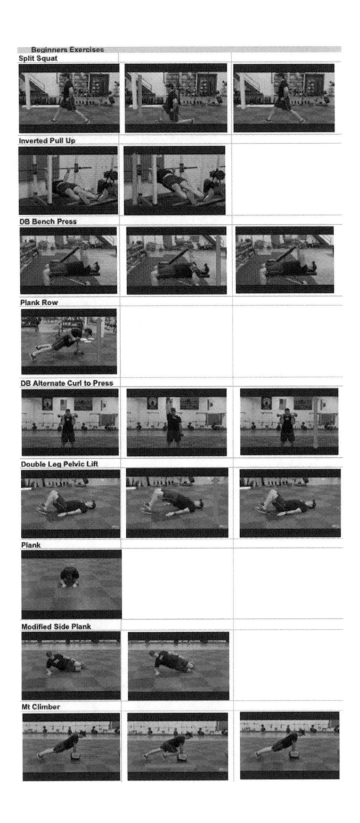

Weight Training Program	
INTERMEDIATE PROGRAM	
Week: 1	

DAY ONE	Instructions: Short Interval Training	
Exercise		

Warm Up: 3 minute Jump Rope + Dynamic Warm Up (see Appendix F)

Cardio: Select any of the following: Running (ie treadmill), Air Dyne Bike, Rowing Machine and Perform the following workout.

Sprint for 30 seconds at Zone 3 (hard), then walk/rest for 30 seconds at Zone 1 (easy) for a total of 20 minutes.
Work to Rest Ratio: 1:1 Intensity: Hard-Easy - once you have completed the cardio portion, move onto the following:
Leg Complex I: Body Weight Squats for 20 Seconds, followed by Squat Jumps for 20 seconds, followed by Squat Holds for 20 seconds, rest 1 minutes.
Perform 3 rounds. **Pull Ups:** 4-5-6-6-5-4 rest 30 seconds between each set: total reps 30 **Push Ups:** 9-9-10-10-11-11-10-10-9-9 reps / rest 45 seconds in between each set: 98 total reps

Cool Down: Walk Easy for 5 minutes and perform static stretching

DAY TWO & FIVE	Instructions: Giant Set: A combination of exercises performed in order with little or no rest in between. For example: Squat, Pull Up, Push Up, Plank......once you have completed a round you start over again.												
Exercise:	Set 1		Set 2		Set 3		Set 4		Set 5		Set 6		Total lbs
	Reps	lbs	Reps	lbs	Reps	lbs	Reps	lbs	Reps	lbs	Reps	lbs	lifted / ex.
1 Lunge	15		15										
2 Inverted Pull Up	15		15										
3 Dumbbell (DB) Bench Press	15		15										
4 Medicine Ball (MB) Push Up	15		15										
4 Plank Row: each side (es)	15		15										
5 DB Alt Curl to Press (es)	15		15										
6 Single Leg (SL) Pelvic Lift (es)	15		15										
7 Stir the Pot (each direction)	5		5										
8 Palloof Press (es)	10 sec		10 sec										
9 Mt Climber (es)	15		15										
Totals	120	0	125	0	0	0	0	0	0	0	0	0	0

DAY THREE, SIX AND SEVEN:	REST DAY (Stratic Strech, Self Myo-Fascial Release Techniques)

DAY FOUR	Instructions: Long Interval Training	
Exercise		

Warm Up: 3 minute Jump Rope + Dynamic Warm Up (see Appendix F)

Cardio: Select any of the following: Running (ie treadmill), Air Dyne Bike, Rowing Machine and Perform the following workout.

Exercise for moderate pace for 1:30 minute at Zone 2- 3 (medium/hard), then walk/rest for 1 minute at Zone 1 (easy) for a total of 25 minutes. Work to Rest Ratio: 1.5:1 Intensity: Hard-Easy - once you have completed the cardio portion, move onto the following: **Leg Complex II:** 20 Body Weight Squats, immediatley 20 split jumps, 10 body weight squats. rest 1 minutes between each round. Perform 3 rounds **Pull Ups:** 4-5-6-6-5-4 rest 30 seconds between each set: total reps 30 **Push Ups:** 9-9-10-10-11-11-10-10-9-9 reps / rest 45 seconds in between each set: 98 total reps

Cool Down: Walk Easy for 5 minutes and perform static stretching

Weight Training Program

INTERMEDIATE PROGRAM
Week: 2

DAY ONE	Instructions: Short Interval Training
Exercise	

Warm Up: 3 minute Jump Rope + Dynamic Warm Up (see Appendix F)

Cardio: Select any of the following: Running (ie treadmill), Air Dyne Bike, Rowing Machine and Perform the following workout.

Sprint for 30 seconds at Zone 3 (hard), then walk/rest for 30 seconds at Zone 1 (easy) for a total of 25 minutes. Work to Rest Ratio: 1:1 Intensity: Hard-Easy - once you have completed the cardio portion, move onto the following: **Leg Complex I:** Body Weight Squats for 20 Seconds, followed by Squat Jumps for 20 seconds, followed by Squat Holds for 20 seconds. rest 1 minutes. Perform 4 rounds. **Pull Ups:** 5-6-6-7-6-6-5 rest 30 seconds between each set: total reps 41 **Push Ups:** 9-10-10-11-11-12-11-11-10-10-9 reps / rest 45 seconds in between each set: 114 total reps

Cool Down: Walk Easy for 5 minutes and perform static stretching

DAY TWO & FIVE	Instructions: Giant Set: A combination of exercises performed in order with little or no rest in between. For example: Squat, Pull Up, Push Up, Plank......once you have completed a round you start over again.

	Exercise:	Set 1 Reps	Set 1 lbs	Set 2 Reps	Set 2 lbs	Set 3 Reps	Set 3 lbs	Set 4 Reps	Set 4 lbs	Set 5 Reps	Set 5 lbs	Set 6 Reps	Set 6 lbs	Total lbs lifted / ex.
1	Lunge	12		12		12								
2	Inverted Pull Up	12		12		12								
3	Dumbbell (DB) Bench Press	12		12		12								
	Medicine Ball (MB) Push Up	12		12		12								
4	Plank Row: each side (es)	12		12		12								
5	DB Alt Curl to Press (es)	12		12		12								
6	Single Leg (SL) Pelvic Lift (es)	12		12		12								
7	Stir the Pot (each direction)	10 sec		10 sec		10 sec								
8	Palloof Press (es)	10 sec		10 sec		10 sec								
9	Mt Climber (es)	12		12		12								
	Totals	96	0	96	0	96	0	0	0	0	0	0	0	0

DAY THREE, SIX AND SEVEN:	REST DAY (Stratic Strech, Self Myo-Fascial Release Techniques)

DAY FOUR	Instructions: Long Interval Training
Exercise	

Warm Up: 3 minute Jump Rope + Dynamic Warm Up (see Appendix F)

Cardio: Select any of the following: Running (ie treadmill), Air Dyne Bike, Rowing Machine and Perform the following workout.

Exercise for moderate pace for 1:30 minute at Zone 2- 3 (medium/hard), then walk/rest for 1 minute at Zone 1 (easy) for a total of 30 minutes. Work to Rest Ratio: 1.5:1 Intensity: Hard-Easy - once you have completed the cardio portion, move onto the following: **Leg Complex II:** 20 Body Weight Squats, immediatley 20 split jumps, 10 body weight squats. rest 1 minutes between each round. Perform 4 rounds **Pull Ups:** 5-6-6-7-6-6-5 rest 30 seconds between each set: total reps 41 **Push Ups:** 9-10-10-11-11-12-11-11-10-10-9 reps / rest 45 seconds in between each set: 114 total reps

Cool Down: Walk Easy for 5 minutes and perform static stretching

Weight Training Program		
INTERMEDIATE PROGRAM		
Week: 3		

DAY ONE	Instructions: Short Interval Training	
Exercise		

Warm Up: 3 minute Jump Rope + Dynamic Warm Up (see Appendix F)

Cardio: Select any of the following: Running (ie treadmill), Air Dyne Bike, Rowing Machine and Perform the following workout.

Sprint for 30 seconds at Zone 3 (hard), then walk/rest for 30 seconds at Zone 1 (easy) for a total of 30 minutes. Work to Rest Ratio: 1:1 Intensity: Hard-Easy - once you have completed the cardio portion, move onto the following: **Leg Complex I:** Body Weight Squats for 20 Seconds, followed by Squat Jumps for 20 seconds, followed by Squat Holds for 20 seconds. rest 1 minutes. Perform 5 rounds. **Pull Ups:** 6-6-7-7-8-7-7-6-6 rest 30 seconds between each set: total reps 60 **Push Ups:** 9-10-10-11-11-12-11-1-10-10-9 reps / rest 45 seconds in between each set: 126 total reps

Cool Down: Walk Easy for 5 minutes and perform static stretching

DAY TWO & FIVE	Instructions: Giant Set: A combination of exercises performed in order with little or no rest in between. For example: Squat, Pull Up, Push Up, Plank......once you have completed a round you start over again.												
Exercise:	Set 1		Set 2		Set 3		Set 4		Set 5		Set 6		Total lbs lifted / ex.
	Reps	lbs	Reps	lbs	Reps	lbs	Reps	lbs	Reps	lbs	Reps	lbs	
1 Lunge	10		10		10		10						
2 Inverted Pull Up	10		10		10		10						
3 Dumbbell (DB) Bench Press	10		10		10		10						
Medicine Ball (MB) Push Up	10		10		10		10						
4 Plank Row: each side (es)	10		10		10		10						
5 DB Alt Curl to Press (es)	10		10		10		10						
6 Single Leg (SL) Pelvic Lift (es)	10		10		10		10						
7 Stir the Pot (each direction)	10 sec		10 sec		10 sec		10 sec						
8 Palloof Press (es)	10 sec		10 sec		10 sec		10 sec						
9 Mt Climber (es)	10		10		10		10						
Totals	80	0	80	0	80	0	80	0	0	0	0	0	0

DAY THREE, SIX AND SEVEN:	REST DAY (Stratic Strech, Self Myo-Fascial Release Techniques)

DAY FOUR	Instructions: Long Interval Training	
Exercise		

Warm Up: 3 minute Jump Rope + Dynamic Warm Up (see Appendix F)

Cardio: Select any of the following: Running (ie treadmill), Air Dyne Bike, Rowing Machine and Perform the following workout.

Exercise for moderate pace for 2 minute at Zone 2- 3 (medium/hard), then walk/rest for 1 minute at Zone 1 (easy) for a total of 20 minutes. Work to Rest Ratio: 2:1 Intensity: Hard-Easy - once you have completed the cardio portion, move onto the following: **Leg Complex II:** 20 Body Weight Squats, immediatley 20 split jumps, 10 body weight squats. rest 1 minutes between each round. Perform 5 rounds **Pull Ups:** 6-6-7-7-8-7-7-6-6 rest 30 seconds between each set: total reps 60 **Push Ups:** 9-10-10-11-11-12-12-11-1-10-10-9 reps / rest 45 seconds in between each set: 126 total reps

Cool Down: Walk Easy for 5 minutes and perform static stretching

Weight Training Program		
INTERMEDIATE PROGRAM		
Week: 4		

DAY ONE	Instructions: Short Interval Training	
Exercise		

Warm Up: 3 minute Jump Rope + Dynamic Warm Up (see Appendix F)

Cardio: Select any of the following: Running (ie treadmill), Air Dyne Bike, Rowing Machine and Perform the following workout.

Sprint for 30 seconds at Zone 3 (hard), then walk/rest for 30 seconds at Zone 1 (easy) for a total of 30 minutes. Work to Rest Ratio: 1:1 Intensity: Hard-Easy - once you have completed the cardio portion, move onto the following. **Leg Complex I:** Body Weight Squats for 20 Seconds, followed by Squat Jumps for 20 seconds, followed by Squat Holds for 20 seconds. rest 45 seconds. Perform 3 rounds. **Pull Ups:** 6-6-7-7-8-7-7-6-6 rest 30 seconds between each set: total reps 60 **Push Ups:** 9-10-10-11-11-12-12-11-1-10-10-9 reps / rest 45 seconds in between each set: 126 total reps

Cool Down: Walk Easy for 5 minutes and perform static stretching

DAY TWO & FIVE	Instructions: Giant Set: A combination of exercises performed in order with little or no rest in between. For example: Squat, Pull Up, Push Up, Plank......once you have completed a round you start over again.												

	Exercise:	Set 1		Set 2		Set 3		Set 4		Set 5		Set 6		Total lbs lifted / ex.
		Reps	lbs	Reps	lbs	Reps	lbs	Reps	lbs	Reps	lbs	Reps	lbs	
1	Lunge	8		8		8		8						
2	Inverted Pull Up	8		8		8		8						
3	Dumbbell (DB) Bench Press	8		8		8		8						
	Medicine Ball (MB) Push Up	8		8		8		8						
4	Plank Row: each side (es)	8		8		8		8						
5	DB Alt Curl to Press (es)	8		8		8		8						
6	Single Leg (SL) Pelvic Lift (es)	8		8		8		8						
7	Stir the Pot (each direction)	10 sec		10 sec		10 sec		10 sec						
8	Palloof Press (es)	10 sec		10 sec		10 sec		10 sec						
9	Mt Climber (es)	8		8		8		8						
	Totals	64	0	64	0	64	0	64	0	0	0	0	0	0

DAY THREE, SIX AND SEVEN:	REST DAY (Stratic Strech, Self Myo-Fascial Release Techniques)

DAY FOUR	Instructions: Long Interval Training
Exercise	

Warm Up: 3 minute Jump Rope + Dynamic Warm Up (see Appendix F)

Cardio: Select any of the following: Running (ie treadmill), Air Dyne Bike, Rowing Machine and Perform the following workout.

Exercise for moderate pace for 2 minute at Zone 2- 3 (medium/hard), then walk/rest for 1 minute at Zone 1 (easy) for a total of 26 minutes. Work to Rest Ratio: 2:1 Intensity: Hard-Easy - once you have completed the cardio portion, move onto the following: **Leg Complex II:** 20 Body Weight Squats, immediatley 20 split jumps, 10 body weight squats, rest 45 seconds between each round. Perform 3 rounds **Pull Ups:** 6-6-7-7-8-7-7-6-6 rest 30 seconds between each set: total reps 60 **Push Ups:** 9-10-10-11-11-12-12-11-1-10-10-9 reps / rest 45 seconds in between each set: 126 total reps

Cool Down: Walk Easy for 5 minutes and perform static stretching

Weight Training Program	
INTERMEDIATE PROGRAM	
Week: 5	
RECOVERY	

DAY ONE	Instructions: Short Interval Training
Exercise	

Warm Up: 3 minute Jump Rope + Dynamic Warm Up (see Appendix F)

Cardio: Select any of the following: Running (ie treadmill), Air Dyne Bike, Rowing Machine and Perform the following workout.

Sprint for 30 seconds at Zone 3 (hard), then walk/rest for 30 seconds at Zone 1 (easy) for a total of 18 minutes. Work to Rest Ratio: 1:1 Intensity: Hard-Easy - once you have completed the cardio portion, move onto the following: **Leg Complex I:** Body Weight Squats for 20 Seconds, followed by Squat Jumps for 20 seconds, followed by Squat Holds for 20 seconds. rest 30 seconds. Perform 3 rounds. **Pull Ups:** 4-5-6-6-5-4 rest 30 seconds between each set: total reps 30 **Push Ups:** 9-9-10-10-11-11-10-10-9-9 reps / rest 45 seconds in between each set: 98 total reps

Cool Down: Walk Easy for 5 minutes and perform static stretching

DAY TWO & FIVE	Instructions: Giant Set: A combination of exercises performed in order with little or no rest in between. For example: Squat, Pull Up, Push Up, Plank......once you have completed a round you start over again.												
Exercise:	Set 1		Set 2		Set 3		Set 4		Set 5		Set 6		Total lbs lifted / ex.
	Reps	lbs	Reps	lbs	Reps	lbs	Reps	lbs	Reps	lbs	Reps	lbs	
1 Lunge	10		10										
2 Inverted Pull Up	10		10										
3 Dumbbell (DB) Bench Press	10		10										
Medicine Ball (MB) Push Up	10		10										
4 Plank Row: each side (es)	10		10										
5 DB Alt Curl to Press (es)	10		10										
6 Single Leg (SL) Pelvic Lift (es)	10		10										
7 Stir the Pot (each direction)	10 sec		10 sec										
8 Palloof Press (es)	10 sec		10 sec										
9 Mt Climber (es)	10		10										
Totals	80	0	80	0	0	0	0	0	0	0	0	0	

DAY THREE, SIX AND SEVEN:	REST DAY (Stratic Strech, Self Myo-Fascial Release Techniques)

DAY FOUR	Instructions: Long Interval Training
Exercise	

Warm Up: 3 minute Jump Rope + Dynamic Warm Up (see Appendix F)

Cardio: Select any of the following: Running (ie treadmill), Air Dyne Bike, Rowing Machine and Perform the following workout.

Exercise for moderate pace for 2 minute at Zone 2- 3 (medium/hard), then walk/rest for 1 minute at Zone 1 (easy) for a total of 18 minutes. Work to Rest Ratio: 2:1 Intensity: Hard-Easy - once you have completed the cardio portion, move onto the following: **Leg Complex II:** 20 Body Weight Squats, immediatley 20 split jumps, 10 body weight squats. rest 30 seconds between each round. Perform 3 rounds **Pull Ups:** 6-6-7-7-8-7-7-6-6 rest 30 seconds between each set: total reps 60 **Pull Ups:** 4-5-6-6-5-4 rest 30 seconds between each set: total reps 30 **Push Ups:** 9-9-10-10-11-11-10-10-9-9 reps / rest 45 seconds in between each set: 98 total reps

Cool Down: Walk Easy for 5 minutes and perform static stretching

YOU HAVE COMPLETED THE INTERMEDIATE LEVEL. GIVE YOURSELF A THE WEEKEND OFF AND RE-TEST YOURSELF.

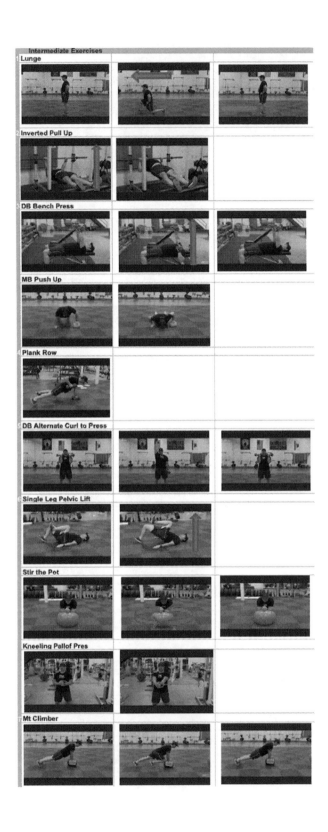

Weight Training Program

ADVANCED PROGRAM
Week: 1

DAY ONE	Instructions: Short Interval Training	
Exercise		

Warm Up: 3 minute Jump Rope + Dynamic Warm Up (see Appendix F)

Cardio: Select any of the following: Running (ie treadmill), Air Dyne Bike, Rowing Machine and Perform the following workout.

Sprint for 20 seconds at Zone 3 (hard), then walk/rest for 20 seconds at Zone 1 (easy) for a total of 20 minutes. Work to Rest Ratio: 1:1 Intensity: Hard-Easy - once you have completed the cardio portion, move onto the following: **Leg Complex I:** Body Weight Squats for 20 Seconds, followed by Squat Jumps for 20 seconds, followed by Squat Holds for 20 seconds. rest 30 seconds. Perform 3 rounds. **Pull Ups:** 7-7-8-8-9-8-8-7-7 rest 30 seconds between each set: total reps 69 **Push Ups:** 10-10-11-11-12-12-13-12-12-11-11-10-10 reps / rest 45 seconds in between each set: 121 total reps

Cool Down: Walk Easy for 5 minutes and perform static stretching

DAY TWO & FIVE	Instructions: Super Giant Set: A combination of exercises performed in order with little or no rest in between. For example: Squat, Pull Up, Push Up, Plank......once you have completed a round you start over again.												
Exercise:	Set 1		Set 2		Set 3		Set 4		Set 5		Set 6		Total lbs lifted / ex.
	Reps	lbs	Reps	lbs	Reps	lbs	Reps	lbs	Reps	lbs	Reps	lbs	
1a Elevated Foot Squat	15		15										
1b Squat Jump	5		5										
2a Inverted Pull Up	15		15										
2b Plank Row: each side (es)	5		5										
3a Dumbbell (DB) Bench Press	15		15										
3b Clap Push Up	5		5										
4 Physioball Punch	15		15										
5a DB Alt Curl to Press (es)	15		15										
5b Spider Push Up (es)	5		5										
6 Physioball Glute Ham	15		15										
7 Stir the Pot (each direction)	5		5										
8 Palloof Press (es)	10 sec		10 sec										
9 Mt Climber with Push Up (es)	15		15										
Totals	125	0	130	0	0	0	0	0	0	0	0	0	0

DAY THREE, SIX AND SEVEN:	REST DAY (Stratic Strech, Self Myo-Fascial Release Techniques)

DAY FOUR	Instructions: Long Interval Training	
Exercise		

Warm Up: 3 minute Jump Rope + Dynamic Warm Up (see Appendix F)

Cardio: Select any of the following: Running (ie treadmill), Air Dyne Bike, Rowing Machine and Perform the following workout.

Exercise for moderate pace for 1:30 minute at Zone 2- 3 (medium/hard), then walk/rest for 30 seconds at Zone 1 (easy) for a total of 20 minutes. Work to Rest Ratio: 1.5:1 Intensity: Hard-Easy - once you have completed the cardio portion, move onto the following: **Leg Complex II:** 20 Body Weight Squats, immediatley 20 split jumps, 10 body weight squats. rest 15 seconds between each round. Perform 3 rounds **Pull Ups:** 7-7-8-8-9-8-8-7-7 rest 30 seconds between each set: total reps 69 **Push Ups:** 10-10-11-11-12-12-13-12-12-11-11-10-10 reps / rest 45 seconds in between each set: 121 total reps

Cool Down: Walk Easy for 5 minutes and perform static stretching

Weight Training Program

ADVANCED PROGRAM
Week: 2

DAY ONE — **Instructions:** Short Interval Training

Exercise

Warm Up: 3 minute Jump Rope + Dynamic Warm Up (see Appendix F)

Cardio: Select any of the following: Running (ie treadmill), Air Dyne Bike, Rowing Machine and Perform the following workout.

Sprint for 20 seconds at Zone 3 (hard), then walk/rest for 10 seconds at Zone 1 (easy) for a total of 24 minutes. Work to Rest Ratio: 1:1 Intensity: Hard-Easy - once you have completed the cardio portion, move onto the following: **Leg Complex I:** Body Weight Squats for 20 Seconds, followed by Squat Jumps for 20 seconds, followed by Squat Holds for 20 seconds. rest 30 seconds. Perform 4 rounds. **Pull Ups:** 8-8-9-9-10-9-9-8-8 rest 30 seconds between each set: total reps 78 **Push Ups:** 13-13-14-14-15-14-14-13-13 reps / rest 45 seconds in between each set: 123 total reps

Cool Down: Walk Easy for 5 minutes and perform static stretching

---

DAY TWO & FIVE — **Instructions: Super Giant Set:** A combination of exercises performed in order with little or no rest in between. For example: Squat, Pull Up, Push Up, Plank......once you have completed a round you start over again.

Exercise:	Set 1		Set 2		Set 3		Set 4		Set 5		Set 6		Total lbs lifted / ex.
	Reps	lbs	Reps	lbs	Reps	lbs	Reps	lbs	Reps	lbs	Reps	lbs	
1a Elevated Foot Squat	12		12		12								
1b Squat Jump	5		5		5								
2a Inverted Pull Up	12		12		12								
2b Plank Row: each side (es)	5		5		5								
3a Dumbbell (DB) Bench Press	12		12		12								
3b Clap Push Up	5		5		5								
4 Physioball Punch	12		12		12								
5a DB Alt Curl to Press (es)	12		12		12								
5b Spider Push Up (es)	12		12		12								
6 Physioball Glute Ham	12		12		12								
7 Stir the Pot (each direction)	12		12		12								
8 Palloof Press (es)	10 sec		10 sec		10 sec								
9 Mt Climber with Push Up (es)	10 sec		10 sec		10 sec								
Totals	99	0	99	0	99	0	0	0	0	0	0	0	0

DAY THREE, SIX AND SEVEN: **REST DAY** (Stratic Strech, Self Myo-Fascial Release Techniques)

DAY FOUR — **Instructions:** Long Interval Training

Exercise

Warm Up: 3 minute Jump Rope + Dynamic Warm Up (see Appendix F)

Cardio: Select any of the following: Running (ie treadmill), Air Dyne Bike, Rowing Machine and Perform the following workout.

Exercise for moderate pace for 1:30 minute at Zone 2- 3 (medium/hard), then walk/rest for 30 seconds at Zone 1 (easy) for a total of 24 minutes. Work to Rest Ratio: 1.5:1 Intensity: Hard-Easy - once you have completed the cardio portion, move onto the following: **Leg Complex II:** 20 Body Weight Squats, immediatley 20 split jumps, 10 body weight squats. rest 15 seconds between each round. Perform 4 rounds **Pull Ups:** 8-8-9-9-10-9-9-8-8 rest 30 seconds between each set: total reps 78 **Push Ups:** 13-13-14-14-15-14-14-13-13 reps / rest 45 seconds in between each set: 123 total reps

Cool Down: Walk Easy for 5 minutes and perform static stretching

	Weight Training Program														

ADVANCED PROGRAM
Week: 3

Firefitnessonline.com

DAY ONE	Instructions: Short Interval Training
Exercise	

Warm Up: 3 minute Jump Rope + Dynamic Warm Up (see Appendix F)

Cardio: Select any of the following: Running (ie treadmill), Air Dyne Bike, Rowing Machine and Perform the following workout.

Sprint for 20 seconds at Zone 3 (hard), then walk/rest for 10 seconds at Zone 1 (easy) for a total of 20 minutes. Work to Rest Ratio: 2:1 Intensity: Hard-Easy - once you have completed the cardio portion, move onto the following: **Leg Complex I:** Body Weight Squats for 20 Seconds, followed by Squat Jumps for 20 seconds, followed by Squat Holds for 20 seconds. rest 30 seconds. Perform 5 rounds. **Pull Ups:** 8-8-9-9-10-10-9-9-8-8 rest 30 seconds between each set: total reps 88 **Push Ups:** 13-13-14-14-15-15-14-14-13-13 reps / rest 45 seconds in between each set: 138 total reps

Cool Down: Walk Easy for 5 minutes and perform static stretching

DAY TWO & FIVE	Instructions: Super Giant Set: A combination of exercises performed in order with little or no rest in between. For example: Squat, Pull Up, Push Up, Plank......once you have completed a round you start over again.

		Set 1		Set 2		Set 3		Set 4		Set 5		Set 6		Total lbs
	Exercise:	Reps	lbs	Reps	lbs	Reps	lbs	Reps	lbs	Reps	lbs	Reps	lbs	lifted / ex.
1a	Elevated Foot Squat	10		10		10		10						
1b	Squat Jump	4		4		4		4						
2a	Inverted Pull Up	10		10		10		10						
2b	Plank Row: each side (es)	4		4		4		4						
3a	Dumbbell (DB) Bench Press	10		10		10		10						
3b	Clap Push Up	4		4		4		4						
4	Physioball Punch	10		10		10		10						
5a	DB Alt Curl to Press (es)	10		10		10		10						
5b	Spider Push Up (es)	10		10		10		10						
6	Physioball Glute Ham	10		10		10		10						
7	Stir the Pot (each direction)	10 sec		10 sec		10 sec		10 sec						
8	Palloof Press (es)	10 sec		10 sec		10 sec		10 sec						
9	Mt Climber with Push Up (es)	10		10		10		10						
	Totals	92	0	92	0	92	0	92	0	0	0	0	0	0

DAY THREE, SIX AND SEVEN:	REST DAY (Static Strech, Self Myo-Fascial Release Techniques)

DAY FOUR	Instructions: Long Interval Training
Exercise	

Warm Up: 3 minute Jump Rope + Dynamic Warm Up (see Appendix F)

Cardio: Select any of the following: Running (ie treadmill), Air Dyne Bike, Rowing Machine and Perform the following workout.

Exercise for moderate pace for 2 minute at Zone 2- 3 (medium/hard), then walk/rest for 30 seconds at Zone 1 (easy) for a total of 20 minutes. Work to Rest Ratio: 1.5:1 Intensity: Hard-Easy - once you have completed the cardio portion, move onto the following: **Leg Complex II:** 20 Body Weight Squats, immediatley 20 split jumps, 10 body weight squats. rest 15 seconds between each round. Perform 5 rounds **Pull Ups:** 8-8-9-9-10-10-9-9-8-8 rest 30 seconds between each set: total reps 88 **Push Ups:** 13-13-14-14-15-15-14-14-13-13 reps / rest 45 seconds in between each set: 138 total reps

Cool Down: Walk Easy for 5 minutes and perform static stretching

Weight Training Program

ADVANCED PROGRAM
Week: 4

DAY ONE	Instructions: Short Interval Training
Exercise	

Warm Up: 3 minute Jump Rope + Dynamic Warm Up (see Appendix F)

Cardio: Select any of the following: Running (ie treadmill), Air Dyne Bike, Rowing Machine and Perform the following workout.

Sprint for 20 seconds at Zone 3 (hard), then walk/rest for 10 seconds at Zone 1 (easy) for a total of 24 minutes. Work to Rest Ratio: 2:1 Intensity: Hard-Easy - once you have completed the cardio portion, move onto the following: **Leg Complex I:** Body Weight Squats for 20 Seconds, followed by Squat Jumps for 20 seconds, followed by Squat Holds for 20 seconds. No rest . Perform 3 rounds. **Pull Ups:** 8-8-9-9-10-10-9-9-8-8 rest 30 seconds between each set: total reps 88 **Push Ups:** 14-14-15-15-16-16-15-15-14-14 reps / rest 45 seconds in between each set: 148 total reps

Cool Down: Walk Easy for 5 minutes and perform static stretching

DAY TWO & FIVE	Instructions: Super Giant Set: A combination of exercises performed in order with little or no rest in between. For example: Squat, Pull Up, Push Up, Plank......once you have completed a round you start over again.

	Exercise:	Set 1 Reps	Set 1 lbs	Set 2 Reps	Set 2 lbs	Set 3 Reps	Set 3 lbs	Set 4 Reps	Set 4 lbs	Set 5 Reps	Set 5 lbs	Set 6 Reps	Set 6 lbs	Total lbs lifted / ex.
1a	Elevated Foot Squat	8		8		8		8						
1b	Squat Jump	3		3		3		3						
2a	Inverted Pull Up	8		8		8		8						
2b	Plank Row: each side (es)	3		3		3		3						
3a	Dumbbell (DB) Bench Press	8		8		8		8						
3b	Clap Push Up	3		3		3		3						
4	Physioball Punch	8		8		8		8						
5a	DB Alt Curl to Press (es)	8		8		8		8						
5b	Spider Push Up (es)	8		8		8		8						
6	Physioball Glute Ham	8		8		8		8						
7	Stir the Pot (each direction)	10 sec		10 sec		10 sec		10 sec						
8	Palloof Press (es)	10 sec		10 sec		10 sec		10 sec						
9	Mt Climber with Push Up (es)	8		8		8		8						
	Totals	73	0	73	0	73	0	73	0	0	0	0	0	0

DAY THREE, SIX AND SEVEN:	REST DAY (Stratic Strech, Self Myo-Fascial Release Techniques)

DAY FOUR	Instructions: Long Interval Training
Exercise	

Warm Up: 3 minute Jump Rope + Dynamic Warm Up (see Appendix F)

Cardio: Select any of the following: Running (ie treadmill), Air Dyne Bike, Rowing Machine and Perform the following workout.

Exercise for moderate pace for 2 minute at Zone 2- 3 (medium/hard), then walk/rest for 30 seconds at Zone 1 (easy) for a total of 24 minutes. Work to Rest Ratio: 1.5:1 Intensity: Hard-Easy - once you have completed the cardio portion, move onto the following: **Leg Complex II:** 20 Body Weight Squats, immediatley 20 split jumps, 10 body weight squats. No rest between each round. Perform 3 rounds **Pull Ups:** 8-8-9-9-10-10-9-9-8-8 rest 30 seconds between each set: total reps 88 **Push Ups:** 14-14-15-15-16-16-15-15-14-14 reps / rest 45 seconds in between each set: 148 total reps

Cool Down: Walk Easy for 5 minutes and perform static stretching

Weight Training Program	
ADVANCED PROGRAM	
Week: 5	
RECOVERY	

DAY ONE	Instructions: Short Interval Training	
Exercise		

Warm Up: 3 minute Jump Rope + Dynamic Warm Up (see Appendix F)

Cardio: Select any of the following: Running (ie treadmill), Air Dyne Bike, Rowing Machine and Perform the following workout.

Sprint for 20 seconds at Zone 3 (hard), then walk/rest for 10 seconds at Zone 1 (easy) for a total of 18 minutes. Work to Rest Ratio: 2:1 Intensity: Hard-Easy - once you have completed the cardio portion, move onto the following: **Leg Complex I:** Body Weight Squats for 20 Seconds, followed by Squat Jumps for 20 seconds, followed by Squat Holds for 20 seconds. No rest . Perform 3 rounds. **Pull Ups:** 9-9-10-10-9-9 rest 30 seconds between each set: total reps 56 **Push Ups:** 15-15-16-16-15-15 reps / rest 45 seconds in between each set: 92 total reps

Cool Down: Walk Easy for 5 minutes and perform static stretching

DAY TWO & FIVE	Instructions: Super Giant Set: A combination of exercises performed in order with little or no rest in between. For example: Squat, Pull Up, Push Up, Plank......once you have completed a round you start over again.

	Exercise:	Set 1		Set 2		Set 3		Set 4		Set 5		Set 6		Total lbs
		Reps	lbs	Reps	lbs	Reps	lbs	Reps	lbs	Reps	lbs	Reps	lbs	lifted / ex.
1a	Elevated Foot Squat	10		10										
1b	Squat Jump	5		5										
2a	Inverted Pull Up	10		10										
2b	Plank Row: each side (es)	5		5										
3a	Dumbbell (DB) Bench Press	10		10										
3b	Clap Push Up	5		5										
4	Physioball Punch	10		10										
5a	DB Alt Curl to Press (es)	10		10										
5b	Spider Push Up (es)	10		10										
6	Physioball Glute Ham	10		10										
7	Stir the Pot (each direction)	10 sec		10 sec										
8	Palloof Press (es)	10 sec		10 sec										
9	Mt Climber with Push Up (es)	10		10										
	Totals	95	0	95	0	0	0	0	0	0	0	0	0	

DAY THREE, SIX AND SEVEN:	REST DAY (Static Strech, Self Myo-Fascial Release Techniques)

DAY FOUR	Instructions: Long Interval Training	
Exercise		

Warm Up: 3 minute Jump Rope + Dynamic Warm Up (see Appendix F)

Cardio: Select any of the following: Running (ie treadmill), Air Dyne Bike, Rowing Machine and Perform the following workout.

Exercise for moderate pace for 2 minute at Zone 2- 3 (medium/hard), then walk/rest for 30 seconds at Zone 1 (easy) for a total of 15 minutes. Work to Rest Ratio: 1.5:1 Intensity: Hard-Easy - once you have completed the cardio portion, move onto the following: **Leg Complex II:** 20 Body Weight Squats, immediatley 20 split jumps, 10 body weight squats. No rest between each round. Perform 2 rounds **Pull Ups:** 9-9-10-10-9-9 rest 30 seconds between each set: total reps 56 **Push Ups**: 15-15-16-16-15-15 reps / rest 45 seconds in between each set: 92 total reps

Cool Down: Walk Easy for 5 minutes and perform static stretching

YOU HAVE COMPLETED THE INTERMEDIATE LEVEL. GIVE YOURSELF A THE WEEKEND OFF AND RE-TEST YOURSELF.

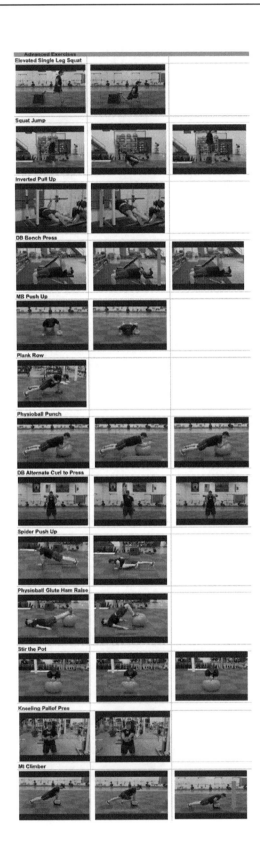

REFERENCES

American College of Sports Medicine (2000). *ACSM's Guidelines for Exercise Testing and Prescription, 6th ed.* Baltimore: Lippincott, Williams, and Wilkins

Bauer, D., et. al. (Oct, 2011). "Cardiorespiratory Fitness Predicts Cardiovascular Risks in Career Firefighters." *Journal of Occupational Environmental Medicine.* 53, 1155–1160

Baur, D., M., Christophi, C.A. Kales, S.N. (2011). "Metabolic syndrome is inversely related to cardiorespiratory fitness in make career firefighters." Journal of Strength and Conditioning Research, 26 (9), 2331-2337

Bogucki, S., and Rabinowitz, P.M. (Oct, 2004). "Occupational health of police and firefighters." Retrieved March 1, 2007, from http://www.harcourt-international.com/e-books/pdf/1024.pdf.

Borg G. (1998). "Borg's Perceived Exertion and Pain Scales." *Human Kinetic,* 63–80

Buchan, D.S., et. al. (2011). "The effects of time and intensity of exercise on novel and established markers of CVD in adolescent youth." *American Journal Human Biology* 23:517–2

Cohen, B.E., et. al. (March, 2012). "Lifetime exposure to traumatic psychological stress is associated with elevated inflammation in heart and soul of body." *Brain, Behavior, and Immunity.*

Eglin, Clare (2007). "Physiological responses to fire-fighting: thermal and metabolic considerations." *Journal of the Human-Environment System*, 10 (1). pp. 7–18

Elliot, D.L., and Kuehl, K.S. (June, 2007). "Effects of sleep deprivation on firefightersand EMS responders." *International Association of Firefighters. 6,* 1–104.

Fahy, F., LeBlanc, P.R., Molis, J.L., "Firefighter Fatalities in the United States."

Findley, B.W., Brown, L.E., Whitehurst, M., Gilbert, R., and Apold, S.A. (1995). "Age group performance and physical fitness in male firefighters." *The Journal of Strength and Conditioning Research,* 9(4), 259–260. Retrieved February 19, 2007, from http://nsca.allenpress.com/nscaonline.

Fernhall, B., and Horn, G. (August 2011). "Firefighting stiffens arteries, Impairs heart function." Illinois Fire Service Institute

Findley, B.W., Brown, L.E., and Whitehurst, M. (2002). "Anaerobic power performance on Incumbent female firefighters." *The Journal of Strength and Conditioning Research,* 16(3), 473-476. Retrieved February 19, 2007, from http://nsca.allenpress.com/nscaonline.

Helgerud, J, et al (2007). "Aerobic high-intensity intervals improve VO_2 max more than moderate training." *Medical Science Sports Exercise,* 39:665–71

Hilyer, J.C., Weaver, M.T., and Gibbs, J.N. (1999). "In-station physical training for firefighters." *Strength and Conditioning Journal,* 21(1), 60–64. Retrieved February 19, 2007, from http://nsca.allenpress.com/nscaonline.

Houmard, JA, et al (2004). "Effect of the volume and intensity of exercise training on insulin sensitivity." *Journal of Applied Physiology,* 96:101–6 International Association of Firefighters (2000). *Death and Injury Survey.* Washington DC, International Association of Firefighters. Retrieved June 2, 2008, from International Association of Firefighters web site: IAFF.org.

Kales, S.N., Soteriades, E.S., Christophi, C.A., and Christiani, D.C. (2007). "Emergency duties and deaths from heart disease among firefighters in the U.S." *The New England Journal of Medicine. 356(12),* 1207–1215

Karter, M. J., Molis, J. (2010). *Firefighter Fatalities in the United States in 2009.* Retrieved April 20, 2011, from www.NFPA.org

Karter, M. J. (2010). *U.S. fire department profile.* Retrieved April 20, 2011, from The National Protection Agency web site.

Karter, M. J. (2006). *Survey of Fire Departments for U.S Fire Experience.* Retrieved June 8, 2008, from The National Protection Agency web site.

Kuehl, K.S., Elliot, D.L., Goldburg, L., and Moe, E. (January 2005). "The Phlame Study: Short-term economic impact of health promotion." *Journal of Investigative Medicine.* 53 (1), 127

Krustrup, P., Mohr, et. al. (2003). "The Yo-Yo Intermittent Recovery Test: Physiological Response, Reliability, and Validity." *Medicine & Science in Sports & Exercise*

Melanson, E.L., MacLean, P.S., Hill, J.O. (April, 2009). "Exercise improves fat metabolism in muscle but does not increase 24-h fat oxidation." *Exercise Sport Science Review.* 37 (2), 93–101

Misner, J. E., Boileau, R. A., Plowman, S.A., Joyve, S., Hurovitz, S., Elmore, B.G., et.al. (1989). "Physical performance and physical fitness of a select group of female firefighter applicants." *Journal of Strength and Conditioning Research.* 3(3), 62–67. Retrieved March 1, 2007, from http://nsca.allenpress.com/nscaonline.

National Fire Protection Agency (2008). *NFPA 1583: Standard on Health-Related Fitness Programs for Firefighters.* Quincy, MA: NFPA. Retrieved June 8, 2008, from The National Protection Agency web site.

National Fire Protection Agency (2007). *NFPA 1582–Comprehensive Occupational Medical Program for Fire Departments.* Quincy, MA: NFPA. Retrieved June 8, 2008, from The National Protection Agency web site.

Orange County Fire Authority. 12, 1–30. Fahs, C. A., Huimin, Y., Ranadive, S., Rossow, et. Al. (April, 2011). "Acute effects of firefighting on arterial stiffness and blood flow." *Vascular Medicine.* 16: 113-118.

Peate, W.F. (2002). "Fitness self-perception and VO$_2$ max in firefighters." *Journal of Occupational and Environmental Medicine,* 44 (6), 546-550. Retrieved February 21, 2007, from EBSCO host MEDLINE database.

Pipes, T.V. (1977). "Physiological responses of firefighting recruits to high intensity training." *Journal of Occupational Medicine,* 19 (2), 129–132. Retrieved February 21, 2007, from EBSCO host MEDLINE database.

Poplin, G.S., et. al. (Oct. 2011). "Beyond the fireground: Injuries in the fire service." *Injury Prevention.* 10

Retrieved June 2, 2008, from www.IAFF.org. Espinoza, N., and Contreras, M. (2007). "Safety and Performance Implications of Hydration, Core Body Temperature, and Post Incident Rehabilitation."

Rhea, M. R., Alvar, B.A., and Gray, R. (2004). "Physical fitness and job performance of firefighters." *The Journal of Strength and Conditioning Research,* 18 (2), 348–352. Retrieved February 19, 2007, from http://nsca.allenpress.com/nscaonline.

Roberts, M.A., O'Dea, J., Boyce, A., and Mannix, E.T. (2002). "Fitness levels of firefighter recruits before and after a supervised exercise training program." *Journal of Strength and Conditioning Research,* 16 (2), 271–278. Retrieved March 1, 2007, from http://nsca.allenpress.com/nscaonline.

Tabata, I., Nishimura, K, Kouzaki, M., Hirai, Y., Ogita, F., Miyachi, M., Yamamoto, K. (1996). "Effects of moderate-intensity endurance and high-intensity intermittent training on anaerobic capacity and VO$_2$ max." *Medicine & Science in Sports & Exercise.* 28 (10): 1327–1330

Takanobu Okamoto, Mitsuhiko Masuhara, and Komei Ikuta (2007). "Combined aerobic and resistance training and vascular function: effect of aerobic exercise before and after resistance training." *Journal of Applied Physiology.* 103:1655–1661

Stone M.H., Wilson, G.D., Blessing, D., Rozenek, R. (Sept. 1983). "Cardiovascular responses to short-term Olympic style weight-training in young men." *Canada Journal of Applied Sport Science.* 8 (3):134–9

Tierney, M.T., Lenar, D., Stanforth, P.R., Craig, J.N., Farrar R.P. (March 2010). "Prediction of aerobic capacity in firefighters using submaximal treadmill and stairmill protocols." *Journal of Strength and Conditioning Research.* 24(3):757–64

University Of Chicago Medical Center (1999). Lack of Sleep Alters Hormones. *The Lancet.*

Made in the USA
San Bernardino, CA
04 January 2017